YOUNG PEOPLE
HEARING VOICES

Young People's Section

THE AUTHORS/EDITORS

Sandra Escher, MPhil, PhD, was a science journalist and worked as a senior researcher at the University of Maastricht, focusing on children hearing voices. She is now an Honorary Research Fellow at the Centre for Community Mental Health, Birmingham City University.

Marius Romme, MD, PhD, was Professor of Social Psychiatry at the Medical Faculty of the University of Maastricht (Netherlands) from 1974 to 1999, as well as Consultant Psychiatrist at the Community Mental Health Centre in Maastricht. He is now a Visiting Professor at the Centre for Community Mental Health, Birmingham City University. His research over the past twenty-five years has focused on the voice-hearing experience.

YOUNG PEOPLE
HEARING VOICES

What you need to know
and what you can do

Sandra Escher
&
Marius Romme

First published 2010
New edition 2012

PCCS Books Ltd
Wyastone Business Park
Wyastone Leys
Monmouth
NP25 3SR
UK
Tel + 44 (0)1600 891509
www.pccs-books.co.uk

Young People Hearing Voices: What you need to know and what you can do

A CIP catalogue record for this book is available from the British Library

ISBN 978-1-906254-57-5

Translated from the original by Bettie Goud
Cover designed by Karin Daniels
Printed by Imprint Digital, Exeter, UK

CONTENTS
Young People's Section

PART 1: WHAT YOU CAN DO IF YOU HEAR VOICES

PART 2: THE STORIES OF EIGHT YOUNG PEOPLE

We dedicate this book to the young people
who took part in the study.

PART 1
What You Can Do If You Hear Voices

Introduction to the Young People's Section: How this book works

This book has mainly been written for children* who hear voices. The information in this book is largely derived from a three-year study amongst 80 children and adolescents who were interviewed about their experiences; children who ranged in age from 8 to 19 years at first contact. Half of them were either undergoing treatment, or had been treated in the past, because of their voice hearing; the other half were not. During the study the voices disappeared in 60 per cent of the children. However, there were also children who did not want to lose their voices.

Little is known about voice hearing in children. Most people still have this notion that it is a disease for life. Based on this view, they are mostly scared of it. In this book, you will find extensive information about how you can look differently at voice hearing; learning to deal with it and tips that might help you to learn to cope with the voices. As a child you are still developing and hearing voices can hamper this development. There is a bit of a bottleneck here, because if you want to recover from the voices, you will need to face up to your development again. Voices give out signals about the problem you have and this could partly be the reason why you are stuck at this point. Voices can provide important information, but they should not control your life. There is more to life than voices.

This book has also been written for parents, teachers and mental health professionals. If they cannot help you with your problem, you will have to face it on your own and that should not be the case.

---

* Throughout this section where the word 'children' is used this also includes young people or adolescents.

There are three parts to this book: two parts on this side for you voice hearers. Part 1 is about what you can do if you hear voices and in Part 2 there are eight stories of children who describe what it is to hear voices. When you turn the book around, you will find Part 3 with information for parents, teachers and mental health professionals.

FOR CHILDREN AND ADOLESCENTS WHO HEAR VOICES

We are asking you for your understanding for the language used in this book. It is impossible to use words that are suitable for all age groups. Our first problem concerns finding the right level of language for all readers; but one single level just does not exist. We have decided to use the word 'child', since it is practical and concise, but also because it conveys a vulnerability. Someone aged 15–18 should not be called a child any more, but we hope that you are not irritated by this word, as you would miss what we have to say. We have chosen to illustrate our text with many examples. The names of the children in the examples are not their real names.

The text will sometimes be too difficult for primary schoolchildren, whereas secondary schoolchildren may find it too simple. If the text is too difficult, please let this be a reason to talk about it to other people, to think about it and to reread it, possibly with someone else. If the text is too simple, please take out the main topic and think about it. Form your own opinion. Talk about it with others you trust.

Recognise what is important – that you accept the voices and you develop a language for your experiences. Only when you have a language for your experiences will they become yours and then you can do something about them. This book is a tool to help you with this. You will probably not finish reading this book in one go. Sometimes we have deliberately repeated things, so that it is possible to understand each chapter separately from the other chapters.

If you have any comments or questions, please email me on: a.escher@skynet.be

's Gravenvoeren, Belgium, August 2010
Sandra Escher and Marius Romme

1

Voice Collective: You're not alone
Rachel Waddingham

In the past year Voice Collective has met lots of young people who hear, see or sense things that other people don't. Although each person has their own unique experience, they have all been relieved to find that they're not alone. Lots of other young people hear voices too.

This chapter comes in three parts. The first tells you a bit about Voice Collective groups and gives you some background to our project. The second shares some of the things we've learned that might be useful to you. The final part gives you a few tips on how to deal with any voices you hear that are difficult or scary.

If you'd like to find out more about Voice Collective, share your own ideas or talk with other young people online – check out our website and peer support forum at www.voicecollective.co.uk. We'd love to hear from you.

ABOUT VOICE COLLECTIVE

In April 2009, funded by Comic Relief and London Catalyst, Mind in Camden launched Voice Collective as a two-year project to develop a London-wide network of peer support groups for teenagers who hear, see or sense things that others don't.

We run these groups in partnership with organisations that are already great at supporting young people. So far, we've set up two groups (one with the Anna Freud Centre and one with The Level: Tower

With special thanks to the children and young people who have taken part in Voice Collective during 2009 and 2010.

Hamlets Young People's Centre). Over the next year we plan to double this.

In the UK at least, our project is unique. An important part of this is that our workers all know what it's like to hear voices too. As project manager, for example, I have seen visions since childhood and heard voices since my later teens. These shared experiences are central to our work.

Since our launch we've seen a real gap between the support people want and the support they often get. We've heard from families across the world who either don't know what help is out there, or are struggling to get the best from it. We also get emails from teachers, youth workers and therapists asking us how best to support the young people with whom they work.

To try and bridge this gap, we act as guides to help young people, families and supporters connect with the information and services they need. We share our experience of coping, recovery and peer support to balance out some of the more negative information people find on the Internet. We also give free advice, support and training where it's needed most (including schools, GPs' surgeries, youth centres and children's charities).

What happens in a group?

Voice Collective groups are a safe space for young people to meet, share their experiences and find creative ways of dealing with them. They offer peer support, not therapy, and are co-facilitated by someone who knows what it's like to hear voices too.

Each group is different. From creating the group rules to deciding what activities to focus on, we work with group members to help make sure they take the lead. So far, groups have included art, drama, games and discussion. To give you a flavour of the kinds of things we talk about, it has included: coping strategies, stigma, strengths and challenges, dealing with doctors and how it feels to be a young person who hears voices.

It's up to each member to choose when, and how, they talk about the voices or visions they have. There's no pressure to focus on them. Sometimes it's enough for people to know that others in the room 'get' what they're going through and won't judge them. The support group members have given each other is fantastic, and much more powerful than what we, as adults, can offer.

Who can come?

Our groups are open to any young person (aged 12–18) who hears voices, sees visions or has any other unusual sensory experience. Often people are struggling with their experiences, but this isn't always the case.

Joining new groups can feel a bit daunting, so we spend time getting to know young people before they come to the group. We look at their support networks, get to know how they cope with their experiences and help them decide whether the group is the right place for them. If it's not, we help them access other support and leave the door open in case they want to try the group some time in the future.

SHARING WHAT WE'VE LEARNED

During the last year we've really listened to what young people have told us about their experiences – what worries them and what helps them the most. Hopefully you'll find something here that makes sense to you. If not, we're always eager to learn more. Why not log onto our peer support forum to share your ideas?

Hearing voices doesn't make you any more different than anyone else

We're all unique in our own way. We all speak, move and understand things differently. If we didn't, the world would really be a dull place. Still, there can be a lot of pressure to just blend in with everyone else. Sticking your head above the crowd and being different can feel like a risk.

If you hear, see or sense things that others don't, you might feel that you're different from your friends. After all, you're having experiences that they're not. The stigma can make things worse – you might worry that you're going 'mad' or be scared of what your friends would say if they knew. It might seem easier to stay away from people altogether, even if you feel lonely and want to talk.

One of the best things about Voice Collective is that it gives people the chance to meet others who have similar experiences. You don't have to hide. It can really help to see that the person sitting next to you doesn't have three heads, a tail or a big label on their forehead – they just happen to hear voices. Over time it gets easier to see that you don't either.

There's more to you than your voices
If you, and the people around you, are really worried about the voices you hear it's easy for them to take centre stage. Sometimes it can seem like they're all anyone thinks or talks about. You might start to feel that everything else about you is either invisible or unimportant. Ignoring the voices completely rarely helps, but neither does focusing all your time and energy on them. It's all about balance.

All of the young people we meet are talented, interesting and unique in their own right. Sometimes they find it hard to see it, though. If, like them, you feel that you're getting lost behind your voices there are lots of things you can do. One of my favourite ways is to create a 'book of you'. Start a scrapbook and use it to draw, write, paint or stick all the things that make you who you are. Include the things you like, your 'pet hates', the people you care about, the things you're proud of – anything and everything you can think of.

Try and see this, or anything else you do, as a work in progress. Keep coming back to it and let it grow and change as you do. Remember that you don't have to do this alone. Your friends and family might have some ideas to add. More importantly, sharing it with them can help them see your strength and individuality as well as the things with which you need help.

Choose what makes you outstanding
Whilst hearing voices doesn't make you weird, strange or 'mad', you don't have to be 'normal' if you don't want to be. It's up to you to decide what makes you special.

In some cultures voices are viewed as a gift. This doesn't mean that the voices are always pleasant or helpful to start with, but that once they are understood and used properly they are an asset. Others believe that voices are linked to creativity or sensitivity. Lots of famous and successful people have talked about hearing voices (from John Frusciante, ex-Red Hot Chili Peppers guitarist, to Ghandi!). Again, the trick seems to be learning how to deal with them. More than this, many people find that the skills and strength they developed to cope with difficult voices have helped them to succeed in other areas of their life too.

Try not to limit yourself. No matter how you view your voices or visions, they are not the only things that can make you stand out. Take some time to see the skills and abilities you already have. Can you hold on to your sense of humour? Do you have amazing attention to detail? Even if you don't see it yet, there really IS something outstanding about you. Get to know your talents and find out how to make the most of them.

Map your support network
Having a solid support network can help you feel confident enough to deal with the problems life throws at you. Some of the young people we meet feel really unsupported and aren't sure where to turn. Others have lots of people trying to help them (family, doctors, therapists and social workers) but aren't getting what they want or need from them.

So, if you think your support network could do with a spot of attention, why not map it out on paper? Draw in all the key people in your life and what kinds of things they help with (from practical problem-solving to helping you chill out or feel safe). Work with someone to look for any gaps or weaknesses in the map. Together, look at ways of filling them. The more you understand about your network, the easier it is to get the right help from the right person at the right time.

Get the best out of professionals and other supporters
Wherever you get your support, it's important that you feel heard and understood. Some of the people we've met have great relationships with the professionals with whom they work (teachers, doctors, nurses and social workers). Others feel that some don't respect, understand or have time for them. In our experience, adults really do want to help but don't always get it right.

If you want someone who supports you to do something differently, why not take the lead? There's no need to wait for them to get it right when you can teach them more about how you're feeling and what does, or doesn't, help. If you want some extra help with this, speak to someone you know who 'gets it' or contact an advocate. The National Advocacy Service, who specialise in helping young people get their views heard, is a good place to start.

In our group, members have found it helps to talk to other young people about their experiences of professionals. Using art and drama, they've come up with different ways of handling difficult situations. These include: making eye contact and looking confident; telling them what words you use to describe your experiences; telling them what you want to talk about; writing down how you're feeling and what you want to happen. Acting these out before you go can help you try out different things and see what works best for you.

Learn what makes you feel safe
Feeling safe is a key part of coping with distress. If you're struggling with voices, visions or other problems in your life there might be times when you feel frightened or vulnerable. As well as feeling horrible, voices and visions often get worse when people are anxious. Finding ways of feeling safe again when you're scared is really important.

Different things work for different people, so it's important to find something that's right for you. You could try: creating a safe corner in a room, filling it with things that help you feel loved and positive; using your imagination to paint a picture in you mind of somewhere you feel safe and relaxed, and keeping a token to help you remember it; using breathing and relaxation exercises.

One of our group members finds that it helps to say seven things that she can hear, seven things that she can see and seven things that she can feel. Little tricks like this help her to put the voices where they belong – alongside everything else she can hear – and make them feel less scary. It's all about taking control.

Tune up your coping strategies
Often, when we meet young people for the first time, they tell us that they don't have any way of dealing with the voices when they stress

them out. I remember feeling like this myself – my voices used to feel very loud and powerful and I felt small and afraid. Still, once we've been working with someone for a while we usually find that they are already doing things to help themselves, even if they don't see it themselves.

The first step to feeling more in control of your life is working out what you already do that is helping. The second is finding ways of building on the best of these, or using them more often. The next step is learning new strategies that help you deal with the things that still bother you. As a starting point, have a look at our website for some coping tips. You might also want to talk to people you know who can cope with stress and see what they suggest.

Learning new coping strategies can be a bit daunting. They can take a bit of time to master, so don't always work straight away. It can help to think of it like learning any other new skill. When you first pick up a guitar you don't expect to be able to perform a solo at breakneck speed, do you? Keep going, try new ways of doing things and be inventive. The more ways you have of dealing with the things that worry you, the more confident you'll feel.

Connect the dots
If you've read the rest of this book you'll already know that lots of young people find that their voices or visions are linked to they way they feel or the things they've been through. Learning how this all fits together can feel a bit like connecting the dots.

Try to treat it like a puzzle – the picture is there, even if you can't see it. At the start the voices might not make a lot of sense and feel totally separate to the way you think and feel. With a bit of help and support, you will be able to work out some of the things that trigger your voices. It can help to write a diary of when you hear them, keeping track of what you were doing, feeling or thinking about at the time.

Once you know more about what's triggering your voices, or what makes them difficult to cope with, the easier it is to find ways of coping with them. The more you feel able to cope, the more confident you'll feel. The more confident you feel, the less you'll be bothered by the things that were triggering your voices.

Take the wheel – live the life you choose

If you've spent a lot of time feeling stressed out or scared by your experiences, you might feel like everything in your life is out of your control. Your parents or supporters might feel really protective of you and, because they're trying to keep you safe and stress-free, might worry about you becoming more independent.

A key part in getting your life back on track is everyone (including you) knowing when it's time for you to take the wheel again. This doesn't mean that you suddenly need to start doing everything yourself. Everyone needs support sometimes. It's more about being able to make choices about your own life and feeling that these are respected. Part of this is about knowing when to ask for help and how to tell people when you don't need it anymore.

Most of all, if you feel that your life has been on hold because of the way you've been feeling – it doesn't have to stay like that. Spend time talking with people about what you want from your life. Reconnect with people you've missed, learn new skills and seek out opportunities. Get the spark back. Sure, you'll makes some mistakes and sometimes you might find you've overstretched yourself, but that's part of life.

Keep yourself safe, tune up your coping strategies, ask for help and learn from things you find difficult. Use your experiences, good and bad, to make you stronger. Hearing voices or seeing visions does not stop you from being a young person. Your life is not over, it's just beginning. Enjoy it.

TIPS FOR DEALING WITH SCARY VOICES

If you're frightened by the voices you hear, the idea of living the life you choose may feel a bit far off. So, in this final section we've put together some tips that can be useful when you're struggling. If you want some more ideas, or would like to share some of your own with us, check out our website (www.voicecollective.co.uk) or peer support forum.

1. Say 'no'

Some people hear voices that tell them to hurt themselves, hurt people they care about or do other things that they don't want to do. This can be really frightening – especially if you think your voices are really powerful or nasty. No matter who the voices say they are, or what they tell you to do, remember that you're in control of your own body. No one has the right to tell you what to do with it.

Saying 'no' isn't always easy – especially at first. You might find that the voices get louder, threaten you or are nasty. Sometimes it helps to think of them as if they're toddlers who are having a tantrum because they're not getting their own way. If no one pays attention, they get bored. If this happens, stay strong. Use some of the coping strategies you already have, or try some of the other ones on these pages. Realising that voices like this are full of hot air is a real step forward.

2. Challenge them

If someone in your life said something nasty about you, you'd probably tell them to stop being mean. You might tell them that they're wrong about you, and say why. It can help to deal with voices in the same way. So, if your voices are saying something you don't like, why not try:

a) Writing a mantra

A mantra is simply a sentence or two that says something comforting that helps you remember what you really think (not what the voices say). If I was hearing a voice that said my mum hates me and is going to poison me, for example, my mantra could be: 'I know my mum loves me. I trust her and know that she would never try to hurt me.'

b) Talking back

If your voices say something that you wouldn't usually accept from someone in your life – tell them that. Tell them, as calmly as possible, that you don't agree with them and that they're being rude. Try not to get into an argument with them. Just say what you want to say and ask them to behave themselves.

c) Getting a second opinion

If you're not sure what to say back to the voices, talk it over with someone you trust. Sometimes writing down some of the things the voices say most often can help. You can think together about some replies, write them down and use them next time you need to.

3. Ignore them

Sometimes challenging your voices can feel too difficult. At times like these, it can be helpful to work on ignoring them. At first, this can take a lot of effort, especially if they are very loud or are saying things that are making you worry. Try writing a list of things you can do to distract yourself or feel more relaxed and keep it with you to give you ideas when you most need them.

As well as trying to take your mind off them, you can try sending them away for a time. Say something like 'I want to watch TV now, I'll speak to you in half an hour'. If the voices try and speak to you it's important to ignore them until the time you've said. When that time arrives, talk to the voices as agreed. This can take a bit of time to master, but it can really work!

4. Use your imagination

Our imaginations can be a powerful tool. Some people are good at imagining sounds, others at dreaming up images. If you have this skill, why not try using it to make the voices seem less scary.

If you can imagine what the voices look like, how could you make them seem less frightening? Would they be as scary if they had a different face, a funny hat or a squeaky voice? What about if they were naughty children, bullies or a bad-tempered, but harmless, old man? Drawing or writing about the voices and using this to change them is a good starting point. Part of their scariness comes from how you think about them, so it stands to reason that if you change how you think about them they'll be less scary.

5. Listen with kindness

This one might sound a bit strange, but if the voices are being nasty you could try treating them with kindness. This doesn't mean agreeing with them, or accepting what they say, but saying 'you must feel really bad to say such nasty things' or 'it's sad that you need to be so mean'. Sometimes, if the voices are saying something that is similar to how you feel, but much more intense, it can help to say 'Yes, I do feel a bit annoyed at my sister – thank you for noticing'.

It can help to see nasty voices as bullies. Bullies have often been through difficult times themselves. Bullying is never OK, but taking the moral high ground can help you feel more in control. It shows you that you have the power to choose how you respond to the voices. They're not calling the shots. Also, if the voices are linked to the way you feel in some way – getting angry with them can end up making things worse.

6. Express yourself

If your voices sound really angry, hurt or distressed it may be a sign that you've got some feelings that you need to let out. Creativity can really help here – especially if you're not sure what you're feeling. Why not try drawing, painting, writing or making something. Close your eyes, take a deep breath and see what happens. Try not to fear the way you feel – there are no good or bad emotions and we need all of them to be healthy. The key is finding ways to express them that don't cause us, or the people around us, problems.

USEFUL RESOURCES

Voice Collective
W: www.voicecollective.co.uk
T: 020 7625 9042
E: info@voicecollective.co.uk

Childline
W: www.childline.org.uk
T: 0800 1111 (helpline)

Young Minds
W: www.youngminds.org.uk
T: 020 7336 8445

National Youth Advocacy Service
W: www.nyas.net
T: 0800 616101 (helpline)
E: help@nyas.net

Headspace Toolkit
W: www.headspacetoolkit.org
E: info@headspacetoolkit.org

Youth Access: For young people's information, advice and counselling
W: www.youthaccess.org.uk
T: 020 8772 9900
E: admin@youthaccess.org.uk

Rachel Waddingham has heard voices and seen visions since her youth. After almost losing herself in the mental health system during her 20s, she feels lucky to have heard Romme and Escher's message of hope and understanding through the Hearing Voices Network. Rachel now works at Mind in Camden as the manager of Voice Collective, a London-wide peer support project for young people who hear, see or sense things others don't. She is continually humbled by the strength and openness of those she works with and would like to thank them for their help in shaping this chapter.

2

What Is Voice Hearing?

What exactly is voice hearing? When you hear voices, what do you experience? If you hear the kind of voices that we talk about in this book, you will hear one or more voices that tell you something, call your name or they may say: 'What are you doing now?' or 'You should not do that' or 'Well done'. These are often short sentences. However, the voice that you hear is not your own voice, but the voice of someone else. In addition, there is nobody near you who says something to you or who could make that sound. Therefore, the most important characteristics of voice hearing are: hearing a voice that is not yours that says something to you while there is nobody near you who says that.

So, how do you know that it is not you? Whenever we asked the children in our study how they know it is not their own voice and not their own thoughts, they would then, for example, answer like this:

> Roger: It's definitely someone else, as I would not say such stupid things.
> Mia: I hear two voices. I cannot be two voices at the same time.
> Nell: I hear a male voice and I'm a girl myself.

When you hear voices, it does not have to happen via your ears. You can hear these voices in different ways, for example, as if they are present in your head. So you will hear them in your head. It could also be as if they come from the outside and you hear them via your ears, but it could also be that you hear the voices in your belly or your chest. The voices can be clear voices, but they could also be whispering voices which the people around you cannot hear.

For example, in the case of Francesca:

> *The voices fall on top of me from nowhere. From the outside, they come inside me via my ears. They come from nearby, but they can also come from the radio or TV or from ghosts that I sometimes see. Therefore the voices come from someone else. I think that other people experience what I experience, but when I ask them they deny this.*

And Sophie:

> *At first I thought the voices came from outside, through the window or the walls via my ears. At that point, they came from a long way away. Now they're inside my head. Moreover, everything that trembles changes into a voice with the beat of that tremble, or it repeats itself within my thoughts.*

Is the experience the same for everyone?

No, absolutely not. Hearing voices is a very personal experience which is different for everybody. However, there are similarities too. The children in our study heard, on average, fewer than five voices. Some heard the voices at night or in the evening, but, like all other children, these children also heard voices during the day. Most of them only heard them in their head, but that is where the similarity ends.

None of the children heard the same voice. The tone of the voice could vary extremely. It could talk in a very loud voice, whisper or talk at the same tone as the people around them. There was also a major difference in characteristics. The voices varied enormously in terms of age; there were male and female voices or those of boys or girls. They could talk in a friendly way or in a very unpleasant, angry or accusing way. On the one hand they could be kind, but on the other hand say very nasty things indeed. Some children heard the voices of ghosts, spirits, cuddly animals, computers or aliens. Some children heard the voices of people they knew, for example, father, mother, brothers, teacher, uncles, aunts, grandfathers or grandmothers. Some children heard a lot of buzzing noises of a crowd of people in a room. All in all, voices could vary enormously.

Miranda hears the voice of a ghost, a human voice, albeit monotonous, sometimes pleasant, sometimes unpleasant.

Monique hears her uncle's voice. This is a very clear, slightly deep, male voice which sounds pretty angry. In addition she hears voices of funny (cartoon) characters.

Wendy hears a furious, angry voice: a 'non-human being'. The tone varies, but is mainly angry.

Paula hears voices of monsters that come inside her via her ears, but they used to reverberate in her head.

Philip recognises the voices. They are all relatives; he hears slightly more male than female voices.

Natalie has been hearing several voices from the age of two and she sees her granddad, shadows, light, light flashes and a girl. At first, it was just her deceased granddad who spoke, who played games with her and who would tuck her in at bedtime so that her mother did not have to do that. Initially she used to hear footsteps too, but she could not see who it was. When it was her granddad, he would say: 'Hello Natalie'.

Some only heard one type of voice, for example, only one male voice whereas others would hear a combination; male, female and children's voices.

Anna hears six voices:, the voice of Jacqueline, an adult woman; of Suzanne, a child about 12 years old; also of Rob and Bernard, two men, and then an unknown man and an unknown woman. The first three she hears on an almost daily basis. The others less often. They are all kind. The latter two, the unknown man and woman, help Anna when she can't solve things on her own.

Polly hears one and, sometimes, two female voices. These are always the same voices of girls around the age of 14 or 15 and they talk in soft voices.

Teresa hears 20 voices of women, men and children.

Patrick hears a good, female voice and a bad, male voice. The woman gives advice, the man interferes and they end up arguing with each other.

In Duncan's case, the voices come in all shapes and sizes. They squeak, growl, sometimes they are high pitched, sometimes they are low pitched. Sometimes the voice comes from a tile and sometimes from the ceiling. One of the voices is quite nice. It is the voice of an army officer who gives orders.

EXTRASENSORY PERCEPTIONS

Hearing voices is called an extrasensory perception, since you perceive something without your senses being used. There are several types of perceptions; not just voices or noises, but you could also see images. More than half of the children saw images too, some smelled certain scents and some others even experienced being touched or saw auras.

George hears voices and sometimes he hears knocking and sees people. He cannot say whether it is a man or a woman. It is usually a kind of shadow. Initially he hears a noise and then he sees something moving. This usually happens in the evening. The shadow whispers or makes a noise by stepping on a branch.

Pete also hears sounds that others do not, like the gate at the stairs which opens and shuts. He hears thumping and squeaking so that it seems there are mice around. At night Pete regularly sees hyenas and lions with long manes and tails. When he experiences this, he also hears voices.

Rachael hears knocking and music. She says: 'It's just as if I'm in a cinema auditorium. The music is loud and thumping. A kind of "house music".'

Barbara has four types of extrasensory perceptions: seeing, hearing, smelling and being touched. She hears noises (murmuring and zooming noises) and sometimes it goes on for a long time. Sometimes a ghost (her voice) touches her. She sees animals being ripped apart with lots of blood around. She smells weed at times when no one else smells it.

A few children saw auras. Auras are colours that hang around people which cannot be seen by everybody. Therefore, there are many different experiences which vary per person.

Sarah has been seeing auras from birth. She has learned to deal with the auras. A psychic has taught her the meaning of the colours. Nowadays Sarah also sees auras around animals and plants.

Laura sees the images of the voices and she sees auras. She started seeing auras about a year before she started hearing voices. According to her, seeing auras is not linked to hearing voices. She can cope with this. When she does not want to see them, or does not want to occupy herself with them, her psychic has taught her how to switch off in her head. The auras are not accompanied by hearing voices, whereas the other visual experiences are.

The fact that you experience these things does not mean that you are crazy, however, you do need to learn how to deal with these experiences, otherwise they will control your daily life and that will make you ill. When you hear voices, it does not mean that they are only negative or angry. More than half of the children also heard positive voices. Since the negative voices bother people, people often only talk about the negative voices.

In our study, we focused on hearing voices only. If you want to read more information about other extra sensory experiences, there is more literature about paranormal psychology, telepathy, clairvoyance and auras. There are bookshops that specialise in this kind of literature. If you are curious about experiences of voice hearers, please read the chapter about the research outcome of the *Maastricht Interview* which is Chapter 5 in the adults' section of this book.

CAN YOU DRAW A CONCLUSION FROM THIS INFORMATION?

For example, if you only hear a few voices, will it be easier for them to disappear? In our study, for 60 per cent of the children the voices disappeared within three years. This was not related to the number of voices they heard. It was important that the child took the initiative in this and learned to deal with the voices. We noticed that the more scared the voice hearers and those around them were of the voices, the more difficult it was to learn how to deal with the experience.

Does the type of voice have an influence on how well you can deal with the voices?

From this study and other studies too, it emerged that the voices were unique like ordinary people, each with their own characteristics. Voices can be pleasant or unpleasant. Therefore, how you deal with each of the voices varies. When you find that a voice says nice things about you or when it protects you, it is easier to deal with than a voice that swears at you and orders you around. About 85 per cent of the children started hearing voices after an event that rendered them emotionally powerless (see Chapter 5). Through their way of talking, their name or their tone, the voices often say something about the people or situations that are involved in these events. It is, therefore, useful to listen to them. We saw that when the voice hearer got more familiar with the voices, the relationship with the voices changed. They could also see positive elements to voice hearing.

What does have an impact?

The frequency, that is, how often they heard voices, had an impact on the continuation of the voices. If people heard their voices very often, it was more difficult to get them under control. Please do not become despondent because of this comment. Various studies have shown that by talking about them in a structured way, the fear of the voices and how often they appeared, decreased.

Is hearing voices only a scary experience?

No, that was not the case. More than half of the voice hearers stated they were hearing positive voices too.

If you are scared of the voices, you are more likely to talk about unpleasant things and the unpleasant voices that cause problems rather than the pleasant voices. Particularly the voice hearers who could not cope emphasised the negative voices and we saw many counsellors do the same. Therapists often focus on the things that are not going well and that is not so surprising as we go to them when things do not go well. Fortunately some therapists also look at and listen to the positive voices and, for example, some use these positive voices to help gain more control over the negative voices.

It could also be the case that voices say exactly those things of which you yourself are afraid. For example: 'You do not have to study for your final exams, as you are too thick to pass them anyway' or 'You might as well not bother, as you won't be able to do that anyway' or 'If I were you, I would put an end to it' or 'You look terrible'. These are all things that you have doubts about and where you feel insecure. Once you realise that it is linked to your own emotions, you can think about it too. For example: what is the likelihood of me failing my exams? Am I studying enough? Do I need help and if so, from whom?

There are voices that are very negative and say things like: 'I would put an end to it'. You should not immediately think about ending your life. It probably means that you cannot see a solution to your problem, but that you do not want to continue like this either. So ask yourself if you have looked at other solutions at all and whether you have put them in some kind of order. Try to come up with five different solutions. Allow others to help you, but you will have to tell them about your problem first of course. Although this might seem impossible, try it as it will help you to feel supported.

If a voice says: 'You look awful' that does not have to mean that you are ugly. It could, for example, mean that the voice thinks that you have neglected yourself and that you need to pay more attention to your appearance.

During the study most children started to think more positively about their voices. Supported by the study, most children found the courage to talk more openly about their voices and their parents were less worried too about hearing voices being a disease.

WARNING

Talking and thinking about the voices might evoke emotions that you find difficult to deal with. Please do not be afraid or put off by that. It is a normal reaction. Voices can often directly or indirectly tell you about problems you have which you think that you cannot solve. It could well be that you are not happy at all with the things they say. However, you do need to realise that every time you experience emotions and the voices react to these and you run away from the voices, you won't be able to learn to deal with them. If you keep on reacting in this way, you will help to keep this problem going and you will not be able to move on from there, which will stop your development.

You are probably thinking: 'Easier said than done …' but that is like giving in and walking away from the problem. If you want to lead your life in a way that means you can like yourself, you will have to do something about that – to face your own anxiety. If you need help, go and find someone who accepts your voices and with whom you can talk about them. Go and find someone who really listens to what you have to say, who thinks it through with you and who can guide you; not someone who tells you he knows how you should deal with your experience as that is something you have to learn by yourself. At the end of the day it is you who has to deal with it, to live with it.

In the study we noticed that most children learned to deal with their emotions and the problems that had led to their voice hearing in a better way. Some were then able to deal with the voices on their own, but most of them were given some help and support. They did not find this in the area of regular mental healthcare, where their voices were not accepted. The next chapter discusses what works and what does not.

3

How Do You Deal with the Voices?

Our study, but also other studies, clearly demonstrates that you can learn to deal with the voices. How do you do that? Since no two experiences are the same, the ways with which to deal with them are not either. It is a very personal thing. What works for one person does not necessarily work for the other. Furthermore, the way you deal with the voices changes over time when you become less scared of them. Moreover, you develop more and more experience and you will get more of a 'knack' for it. In the third year none of the children in the study dealt with their voices in the same way as in the first year. It was striking that they took the initiative far more and, because of that, gained more control.

Looking at it more closely, learning to deal with voices actually means learning to deal with gaining control. How do you describe control? Simply put, control means being able to play a part in deciding what you are going to do. However, control does not come easily; you need to make an effort. You need to fend for yourself and then know what you want. There are only very few people on this earth – or perhaps nobody at all – who has total control over their own life; not even the Queen! Being in control means being able to say 'yes' or 'no' to things in your everyday life. However, 'yes' or 'no' sounds rather 'all or nothing', but that is usually not the case. Between 'yes' and 'no' there is room for negotiation. An example: if your mother wants you to go to bed at 9.30pm or that you do your homework now and you do not agree with her, try and keep having a say in things by saying: '10pm is OK too, isn't it?'; or 'Please can I watch the end of the film? It is so gripping' or 'I will do my homework as soon as I've finished playing this computer game.'

In order to get an idea that you have a say in things too, you need to learn to negotiate: learning to reach a compromise. If you cannot reach a compromise, you will find dealing with your voices even more difficult.

Of course, it is difficult to negotiate with your voices about control, about what you want. After all, you never asked for these voices. They are uninvited guests and gatecrashers in your head. They often have no manners. They can swear, make a racket, they blackmail you or give orders – in short, controlling your life or having too much influence.

If you do not want to live like that, you will have to decide for yourself that you are going to do something about the voices. The same applies when you are being bullied at school. If you let that happen and you do not defend yourself, they will bully you even more. Something positive will happen only when you show where you draw the line. You may have to get someone else involved who can help, or enrol in a self-defence course or think of something else. The longer you delay telling the other person he has overstepped the line, the more difficult it becomes to reverse it. The control of the voices grows, whilst your feeling of powerlessness grows at the same time. Voices will not state modestly: ' Ho, ho, not so much'. They will grab as much as they can and as much as you will allow them. Voices will go on until you have determined your attitude towards them. That is their challenge to you: to dare you to develop.

You need to realise that voices are not like normal human beings with a normal body and hands and feet. It is more as if they come from another world, a mental world, the world of feelings. In Chapters 6 and 7, we will look more closely at the link between voices and feelings. Here we will discuss the problem of the control the voices have.

Since they do not have any hands and feet, they cannot really do anything for real in our world. At most they can use you, they only have suggestive control. If they want you to do something, they will order you about as they cannot do it themselves. It is always your choice whether you do as they tell you to or not. The control that they have over you is only the control that you yourself give them.

How do you deal with that? It is useful to listen to what they have to say, since they can also say very sensible things. However, you will have to think about whether you find that they are saying good things or not. You can and must decide for yourself to do or not do what they ask of you.

Children who get on well with their voices do not really experience this control problem, as they deal with the voices as they would with a wise friend or wise granddad or granny. They listen to the voices and then think about the things they said. Their voices often give very sensible advice and they never ask them to do strange things. For example, they might advise: 'Why don't you wear these black shoes, as they go much better with the red skirt?' or 'If I were you, I would start my homework now, otherwise you will never finish in time'. So these are things that you can easily do. It is not a matter of control, but more like friendly support.

Control often causes a difficult problem: it leads to disputes and abuse of power. Power develops the moment there is inequality in a relationship. If you have power, it does not mean that you can simply do everything that you think is right. That is abuse of power. Examples of people who thought they could do anything they liked are scattered through history, such as dictators like Sadam Hussein and, further back, Hitler and Stalin. Abuse of power shouldn't happen between people. Voices shouldn't abuse their power either.

Enough about this theory, what should you do?

WHAT DID THE CHILDREN IN THE STUDY SAY ABOUT DEALING WITH THE VOICES?

We asked them: 'What do you do when you hear voices?' The techniques mentioned by these children varied in terms of their success and some worked better for one child than another.

Finding distraction

Thirty-three children said, 'When you find distraction, you transfer your attention from the voices to something else. For example, you read a book, watch a film, listen to music or whatever else. It is about doing something you like. Something you can easily concentrate on.' I can, for example, imagine that a computer game takes up all your attention.

Banishing voices

A number of children mentioned banishing the voices as a coping strategy. For some children this worked so well that, indeed, the voices stayed away completely. Those children could also get really angry at the voices. The anger had to come from deep inside them so they could really feel it.

When you are still really scared, it is difficult to be convincingly angry. In this case it is better to banish the voices temporarily. For example, you can tell them: 'Why don't you come back at 4pm when I am in my room at home?' Make sure that you are there at that time. You need to take your voices seriously and stick to your promises. When you do that, you will notice that they will get angry less easily.

Ignoring voices

Twenty-eight children said, 'You just pretend not to hear them.'

Not listening to the voices

If you are still really scared about what is happening to you because you are hearing voices, you may even be too scared to listen to the voices. If you do that, the fear will cause it to go on.

Listening to the voices

For some children it helped to listen to the voices. They decided for themselves whether what the voice said was to their benefit or not. We know two girls who were given advice by the voices on how they should dress. One of them remained critical. When the voice advised her to wear red shoes and an orange dress, she would not do that. The other girl did as the voice told her. She said: 'He wants me to just wear black clothes and I don't even like black.'

If the voices say things you do not like, you can decide not to listen to them any more. We know children who told their voice; 'I will listen to you again when you tell me something useful'.

You should not always take the things the voices say literally. Voices often talk by way of metaphors. When the voice says: 'She is making a mess of it again' it could be that the voice means that you are making a mess of your life because you are not making the most of the chances you get.

Besides, not all voices tell the truth anyway. Some voices pretend to know everything as if they are almighty, but when you look into that, it is not true at all. Therefore, if you think that whenever the voices say something, they are right, you give them power they do not deserve if you don't even ask them to prove what they say is right. After all, the voice needs to show that he is reliable too if he wants you to listen to him.

Talking to the voices

You can talk to the voices. Not all voices want this, but there are voices that really like it since they can explain to you what they are doing. We know a girl with an aggressive voice that said: 'Just put a end to it'. When she asked the voice what he meant, he explained: 'If you are not doing anything with your life, you might as well put an end to it.' It was well-meant advice, but said in the wrong way.

There are different ways in which you can talk to the voices. You can call on the voices and you can ask them a question yourself, talk to them about things that matter to you or ask them for advice. You can also start talking to them when you start to hear them and respond to what they are saying. The benefit of the former is that you choose the moment that you want to talk. That is power. You decide when you do something.

If you do not dare to start a conversation, why don't you listen to what the voice says and answer 'yes' if it is true and 'no' if it is not true. If you still do not dare to listen, you may have to look for a place where you feel safe; for instance, when you lie in bed with your cuddly toys. If you do not dare to do it when you are alone, why don't you sit with someone your trust, like your mother.

Children who were receiving help called on the voices less often. That could have been caused by the fact that the emphasis in treatment had been less on dealing with voices, but it could also have been that these children remained scared of their voices.

Doing something else

If you start hearing voices when doing your homework, you can take a brief time out and do something else. You can walk to the fridge and get yourself something nice to eat; go to your mum and ask her something that has nothing to do with voices; hug your dog or go to the loo. There are many things you can think of that you can do. The idea is to take a little break.

Visit or phone someone
A number of children visited someone when the voices were being a nuisance, for example, a friend or they would phone someone like their granny or granddad. The idea is that you get this feeling that there is someone else around that you care about and they care about you, that you are not alone. It would be really good if you know another voice hearer, as you could ask for advice or share your experiences.

Shutting yourself off from the voices
There were children who could shut themselves off from the voices by, on the face of it, building a kind of screen around themselves. For example, this can be a circle of roses or an imaginary wide coat around your shoulders. Shutting yourself off is a technique that is used by people with paranormal powers when they want to shut themselves off from the emotions of the people around them. They also do that, for example, in a department store where too many people are moving around with too many different emotions or when they enter a party venue. It is simply learning to protect yourself.

Keeping a diary
There were children who liked keeping a diary. Some wrote about the things the voices said, others just about the things that happened to them during the day and not about the voices. Another group only started writing when the voices appeared and they would continue to write regardless of what the voices were saying. How did the voices react? Some voices do not mind these diaries at all, but there are voices that do not like them. Some children wrote in spite of the fact that the voices objected. You need to find out for yourself, what you dare to do and how your voices react.

There are also children who think up a method of their own
For example, a boy heard two voices of metal men. He had started hearing them after he came round from a general anaesthetic. This boy drew the two metal men in doctors' coats, drew an injection needle

and fantasised that he was giving the two men an injection. It worked as the voices disappeared.

Another boy made a computer game with a labyrinth in which the voice would circle. He, himself, was a round ball with a large mouth, which could eat the voice. We also know a child that started to pray and it worked.

Some therapists are very creative. On the advice of her therapist one girl locked her voices in a cage and she then threw away the key. Together with her therapist she threw away the cage. There was a girl who put the voices in little black men which she threw out of the window. Another girl saw little fat men who told her nasty things. She washed the black men so they became white and she was no longer afraid of them.

WHEN YOU LEARN TO DEAL WITH THE VOICES, THE FOLLOWING THINGS ARE IMPORTANT

Doing something or nothing

We have given you all kinds of examples of children who would do something when they heard voices. There are also children who do nothing and feel overwhelmed by the voices. If you do nothing, it is easier to lose yourself in listening to your voices. Dealing with voices, that is, deciding that you will do something about it, is a way of protecting yourself against the power of the voices. You feel less overwhelmed by them. You come to realise that you have power too.

Voices challenge you and this challenge is to develop yourself: learning to deal with things that scare you and you don't know how to deal with. Learning to live in a society that is not very friendly, taking responsibility that befits your age, for example, taking on a household chore such as walking the dog, doing the dishes or agreeing to do something your parents ask you to do.

Of the children in the study, about 85 per cent started hearing voices as a result of a trauma. A trauma is something that other people do to you, that you did not want, that you cannot cope with, that makes you feel powerless. The voices challenge you to find the answer to a problem; to find your own power to do something; to rediscover your own power; to demand your place, receiving recognition of your problem.

Overstepping the limit

It regularly happens that because of the voices children are overstepping limits, as in the case of George, who was chasing his little brother around the house with a knife; or Miranda, who stole her mother's debit card, took out £600 and spent it; or Thea, who told her parents she needed a mobile phone in order to deal with the voices. She subsequently landed her parents, who were on a low income, with monthly phone bills of £800.

There are all sorts of things that may have happened in your past, but when you do things like that, you have to ask yourself whether the things you do help you gain control of your life. You remain responsible for your own behaviour. Perhaps you can think of something upon which you are able to vent your anger and powerlessness that does not damage other people. For example, you can get it out of your system by thumping a pillow or ball really hard or by looking for physical discipline in a sport. Some children did exactly that: Pete noticed that he was good at cycling, Jasmin was good at swimming and Alfie at football. All three started taking part in matches and started training for these. The discipline of sport was very useful in learning to deal with voices. If you vent your frustration on others in an uncontrolled way, as that is what it often boils down to, eventually you will lose the support of your parents. Whatever you think of them right now, they can help you get out of this situation. Please do not make unnecessary enemies. Teach people around you how they can help you.

Fear

Learn to deal with your fear. Voices can have power, but that also applies to fear. Fear has its own power. Fear can have control over all your emotions. Fear can lead to you feeling powerless, thinking that you cannot do anything any more.

If you are scared, this can lead to all kinds of mental and physical reactions too. For example, you are not able to think clearly any more, get dizzy, start to sweat, feel sick, feel that your face turns as white as a sheet. These are normal reactions to fear that also happen to people who get scared but do not hear voices.

Voices cause different reactions – making you confused, taking over your thoughts, making so much noise that you cannot hear others any more, irritating you so much that you get angry, cracking jokes that make you laugh out loud so that people around you think you are crazy. You really should ask yourself, what is worse: the fear or the voice? In our study we saw that many children were scared in the first year. When the fear diminished, they were able to deal with the voices in a better way. It is complicated, as the fear and the voices are linked, but not everything you feel is caused by the voices. It could also be your body responding to fear by getting hot and sweating, or the opposite, by becoming very cold.

SUMMARY

Dealing with voices is a process in which you have to find a balance with the voices. In this process, you will be challenged to your limits. If you do not accept the voices, you will continue to have to fight and you will not succeed in defeating them. You will then spend all your energy on the rejection rather than thinking about what you do and do not want. You will have an aggressive relationship with them and that is never helpful.

If you want to deal with the voices five things are important:

1. accepting the voices
2. deciding that you want to learn how to deal with them
3. using your own creativity to see what suits you best
4. having strength of mind
5. change your relationship with the voices. Become interested and friendly to them. Listen to what they are trying to tell you
6. regaining power and learning to impose limits on the voices

4

What Kind of Influence Do the Voices Have?

In this chapter, you will find new information, as well as repetition from other chapters. We found that this was unavoidable. Although we differentiate between elements such as influence and fear in the *Maastricht Interview*, they cannot really be separated that clearly as they are mostly interlinked. We differentiated them from each other as it provides structure. If you keep on dumping them in the same pile, you will never get good insight into them. It is, for example, good to discover what comes first: the fear or the voices, or is it the other way around? It could be that the voice scares you by what it says to you or it could be that your body reacts to the fact that you are hearing voices and that you have not accepted that yet.

This chapter covers:

- positive and negative influence of voices
- influence of the voices on fear and anger
- influence of the voices on your thoughts
- blackmail and compulsive actions
- whether the voices are always right

CHANGES

We would like to stress again that the influence of the voices will almost always change over time. If you are having a bad time with your voices, you may think that it will always be like that. That is not true. The voices change, but it helps if you become more active yourself. Sometimes you may not notice that things have changed. We spoke to parents who told us that hardly anything had changed, but at the same time they gave us examples of things that had changed, things that their child was doing differently now; for instance, not watching television on his own in his bedroom, but instead going with his parents to a birthday party. The parents were not aware that their child had changed. They were too focused on everything that was going wrong. They had got into that habit.

The majority of children (80 per cent) were scared of the voices in the first year and that fear prevented them from accepting the voices and learning how to deal with them. As early as the second year this had changed in many of them. Only 50 per cent of the children continued to be very scared of the voices. For those who remained scared and who did not learn how to deal with this fear, the voices disappeared less quickly.

INFLUENCE

Whether you like it or not, voices can have quite a lot of influence on your life. The fact that something or someone has influence on you cannot be avoided. Just think about the situation at home; what happens between you and your parents, your sister, your brother or your friends. If you see or phone each other regularly during the day, you will always have an influence on each other; for example, if your sister says that it is not very cool to read a Harry Potter book, she might spoil your reading pleasure. The fact that someone has an influence on you does not have to mean that that is only something negative. People can also have a positive influence on your life and they can, perhaps, influence you to keep going with something, or they may give you advice on your sport or simply have an influence on your mood. By giving you a present, somebody can make you happy.

Being influenced does not have to be a bad thing, but you must be careful that someone does not try to have too much influence, since then your own 'I', your own true self, will disappear. You will not know what you want any more. If, for example, your mother interferes with everything you do – the clothes you want to wear in the morning, what you put in your packed lunch, what and how much you eat in the evening, how long you are allowed to talk to your friends or phone them – commenting on everything you do and say, because it is not good enough, etc., she may mean well, but it will lead to too many rules and may make you feel insecure and lacking in confidence.

Someone else can help you maintain structure in your day and life, but he or she should not think they can decide what you think. This applies to voices that want to control what you do too, as then it will feel like they take over from you, which means you will lose your own 'I'.

How does the influence of voices happen?

There are many ways in which too much influence can develop. For example, when there is too much contact. If the voices are present regularly and they are a pain, it is more difficult to stick to your own opinions.

The voices can also gain influence by the emotions they evoke. They can scare you, make you angry or sad when they demand things of you and force you to do things that do not fit with your personality like stealing, hitting people or picking fights. They can also try to make you do things by blackmailing you.

The voices can evoke emotions, but they can reinforce them too. For example, they can make you so angry that you do something that is not very clever. We know a lovely girl who had to queue at the checkout in the supermarket for a long time. Initially she became impatient, then angry and then she started to hear voices that made her even angrier. She got so angry that she drove the trolley into the woman in front of her really hard, so hard, in fact, that this woman fell over the trolley. The girl said the following about this incident: 'I did it to regain control of the voices'. It sounds like a good excuse, but if you do something like that, you hurt someone else. There are other ways to regain control, for example, by telling the voices that you will give them attention once you have left the shop.

The voices can make you powerless, so powerless that you do not do anything any more, that you believe they will keep you under their control and you completely surrender yourself to the voices. Both examples deal with extremes. Many children didn't let it go that far and were able to find a balance. They learned how to deal with the voices in their own way. That is how they remained in control (see Chapter 3).

The voices have an influence when they can convince you that they know more than you, as if they know everything, that it seems as if they are in control. If that happens, it is best to talk to the voices and ask them how they know all these things. Some voices are speechless when they are asked questions. You will notice that they mostly do not know the answer and that they are bluffing.

Positive influence

What kind of influence did the children in the study describe? Let's start with the positive kind. It is usually assumed that voices are only negative and that is not true. Voices are far more positive than people who do not know much about them assume. The things that are known about voice hearing mainly come from the world of psychiatry – and that is not fair. In psychiatry you mainly see people who have serious problems with voices and who cannot cope with them. Voice hearers who end up in psychiatry have been made powerless by the voices. These are people who have not yet learned to trust their own strengths. If therapists were only to see those people who cannot deal with them, they would not exactly get a positive image of voice hearing. However, from various studies we now know that voice hearing is apparent in 8% of children in the general population and most voice hearers are not looking for psychiatric help since they have learned how to cope based on their own strengths. We are not saying that looking for help is a bad thing, but we do say that, at the end of the day, you have to do it yourself. You cannot go and see a therapist, hand over your voices and tell him 'Please deal with this for me'.

Of the children in our study, 50 per cent heard both positive and negative voices. These positive voices could reassure: 'Don't get so angry, as it won't help you at all' or give advice like: 'I would wear the red shoes, they look a lot nicer' or 'I would do my homework now, you may not have time for it later'. The voice told a boy who was bullied by a classmate in the schoolyard during lunch break: 'Why don't you climb to the very top of the climbing frame, as he won't dare to follow you there?' That was true; the bullying boy did not dare to climb to the top. There were several voices that gave warnings while out on the road: 'Why don't you get off your bike here, as a dangerous car is about to come around the corner?' It might have been a good warning, but it made the children more insecure in traffic.

We noticed that the voices would mostly first appear to protect someone: in situations where things were difficult at school, at times when the children had to prove that they had understood the things they had been taught. There were voices which gave advice during a test, but there was often a catch in it somewhere. The voices remained positive as long as the children did not listen to them too much. If children listened to them more often they became dependent on the advice of the voices and, for example, they would not study for a test any more. But it was at that point that the positive voice changed into a nasty, awful voice that demanded attention.

Changes

You have to realise that the influence of voices usually changes over time. The influence today is not the same as the one next year. By getting to know your voices better, by learning to talk about them and thinking about them, their influence reduces. You notice that as they occur less often, you are less scared of them too.

It often happened that people thought that nothing had changed and that is because our memories don't want to cooperate. We prefer to forget unpleasant things. So how will you know whether things change over time? The easiest way is to keep a short diary. In our study we noticed changes because we interviewed the children about their voices four times with a year in between and then compared the four interviews with each other.

YOUR OPINION ABOUT THE VOICES

It also became apparent that the influence of the voices was linked to the children's attitude towards the voice, that is, with what the children associated the voices. We will explain this here. Voice hearing can be nice if the voice is linked to something nice. Caroline heard a voice, called Vie. Vie meant 'life' to her. Vie stimulates her to live. Caroline: 'When I am swimming, then I have Vie there as my personal trainer. She encourages me.' Furthermore, the voice sounded like the voice of her granny, who had passed away not long before. For Caroline, hearing voices was not something of which she was scared.

Emma heard a voice that was sometimes positive; for example, when she had a flat tyre, the voice advised her to take another route where there was a phone booth, so that she could phone her parents. Although she was scared of the voice, she dared to listen to his advice.

For Peter the voice was linked to both fear and powerlessness which led to physical reactions. There was nothing positive about the voice according to him. As soon as he heard the voice, he got scared and he did not dare to listen to him.

If you react like that, you get stuck. If you do not hear what the voice says, you cannot think about what the voice is saying and what kind of meaning that could have. For example, when a voice does not allow you to go outside alone, it could well be that being outside is not safe for you, since there are children who make the neighbourhood an unsafe place. If the voice warns you, it may be a good idea to start thinking about how you can make things safer for yourself. You could take your mobile with you, or your dog, a cuddly toy, a friend or make sure you are home before it gets dark, or you could even do a course in self-defence.

If a voice talks about dying, it may mean that he wants you to change, that you should start a new life. You should start thinking about the things you do not like in your life right now and how you think you can change your life and who can help you. You should not stop living because of the word 'death', nor should you become scared of it and do nothing about it.

Here is another example about the influence of the meaning for someone. This is an everyday example. We took a voice hearer to the station where there was a carnival band playing very loudly. At that moment, I was not in the mood for all this cheerfulness and I found the music awful. Even worse it gave me a headache. The voice hearer had a totally different perception. He shouted very enthusiastically: 'Fantastic, they are here to see me off!' The world is a much nicer place if you give a positive twist to things that happen to you. It makes life a lot more pleasant. Why don't you try it, you have nothing to lose.

The influence of the voices is not a total package, it comes with a dosing spoon and you are the one holding it. It is something that requires you to make your own decisions. You cannot just blame someone else for too much influence. You are involved too. The level of influence that you will allow another person to have depends how confident you feel, what you dare to do. There were children in the second and third year of the study who very convincingly told the voice, 'Forget it, I want nothing to do with you any more'. In that way they did not allow the voices too much influence. If you start feeling scared and you do not do anything about it, the influence will increase automatically.

We noticed that the nuisance the voices caused was often made the focus of attention and, as a result, it was forgotten that not all voices were negative and that positive voices can help you with problems and that you can also learn how to deal with negative voices.

INFLUENCE THROUGH FEAR

Let's talk about fear again here. In the study we noticed that fear was the main offender. Fear determined the influence of the voices. Two boys even got so scared of the voices during the study's interviews that they showed physical reactions. They became very pale, felt cold and one of them started to sweat. Both boys were courageous and decided not to be terrorised in this way by the voices. They continued to take part in the study. The mothers of both boys decided they needed help and they looked for therapy outside the area of regular healthcare. Both were taught by an alternative therapist to discover a language for their experience and to talk about it more often and in a better way. They learned not to lock up this fear within themselves but, on the contrary, to bring it out in the open by way of words. That did a lot of good, but there is a condition – you need to make a decision. You have to decide to keep going in order to learn how to deal with your fear. If every time you are scared you stop, fear will get a grip on you. If you are very scared and you still want to continue, you will have to find someone or something that makes you feel safe. For example, hold your mother's hand. If you do not like doing that, I am sure you can think of something else yourself. Please don't just give up after one try. Keep on trying for at least a week.

Voices can forbid you to talk about them to others and they will threaten you with punishment if you do it anyway. They make a secret of themselves. Why do they do that? The things I am going to say now may sound a bit strange and you may have to read it again or talk about it to someone, but in our study this mainly happened when the voices had not been accepted. It may sound strange, but most voices want to be accepted, appreciated and not be ignored. Most voices have a message; they talk about something with which you have problems. If you do not understand the voices, they feel rejected and they get angry and make you feel scared. At that point, you are in a fight with them and all the stories suggest that being in a fight with the voices is not going to help you.

Fear can ruin the pleasure you get from things you enjoy. The voices liked doing that. When Paula was watching a TV quiz and she was enjoying herself, the voice would say: 'If you do not answer ten questions correctly, I will scare you'. He ruined her enjoyment of the quiz. Paula would then walk away from the TV and the voice would punish her by showing her scary skeletons at night. Since she knew that the voice would do that, she did not dare to go to bed. She told her dad, who offered a good suggestion; he would check under her bed every night for skeletons. If he did not see them, Paula would go to bed reassured.

In Suzanne's case the voices would ruin her pleasure in drawing. 'When I am drawing something, they will say: "That looks awful. It is a shit drawing", and when they say things like that, I just stop, as I do not feel like drawing anymore.' Later, when Suzanne felt more in control of the voices, she did not care at all about these remarks any more.

When you are scared, for instance, in the dark or when going to bed, and you cannot solve this on your own, you need other people's help. What kind of help works? Let's start by saying what does not work. That is the kind of help where the other person takes over your responsibility. In the study parents would say that when their child was very scared at night, they would let the child sleep with them in their bed but, then, they could not sleep either any more and, therefore, their child's fear gradually became a family problem as the entire family suffered from lack of sleep.

An extreme example. A father told us that his daughter, Vera, had been sleeping in between him and his wife for the last four years. Vera had got used to it so much that she started causing problems when her parents wanted to go away for a weekend. Vera would not have it, as she would want to join her parents. No aunt or uncle were good enough to replace her parents. If Vera's strategy had indeed worked, that might have been OK, but no, Vera started suffering more and more from the voices and she started demanding more and more. Her father noticed that Vera always felt cold. Halfway through the night she would pull the duvet over her body even further and make herself even more comfortable. In those four years Vera had grown quite a bit and her father had ended up on the edge of his own bed feeling cold without his duvet. He did not dare to say anything about this as there was no reasoning with Vera and everything was blamed on the voices. The parents claimed that the voices also influenced their lives.

Things that worked well: we noticed that it helped if parents set their own limits, but at the same time taking the voices seriously. For example, the voices told Iris to pray for such a long time before dinner that the food was getting cold. After having eaten several cold dinners, her parents said: 'You can go and pray in the corridor for as long as you like. We want to eat a warm dinner.' That agreement worked well for both Iris and her parents. Such an agreement can only work if you both really want it. Sometimes it may take a little while before you find out what works best. You have to keep going and be patient and that is often the problem.

There are also parents who handled things in a different way than the father who checked every night under the bed of his child to see if there was something underneath it or not. Some parents switched on a little corridor light or they kept the door ajar. Some parents told their children that it was OK to call for them, but only twice per evening at most, certainly not more often, etc. A few older girls had another solution; they took their boyfriend to bed.

Apart from the voices, what else scared the children?
They were: scared to be alone; scared of burglars; to go to sleep; to go to the loo in the dark at night along the dark corridor; to walk outside alone in the street; of people who were walking behind them; to go to school; of scary posters; of the haunted house, etc. All kind of things that everybody is scared of, some more than others.

INFLUENCE ON ANGER

It happens often that the voices make you angry. That anger is very understandable as the voices enter your head without being invited and do not seem to want to leave. They want to be in control of your head. You need to be really dim to let that all happen to you.

It was interesting that when the voices made someone angry, we noticed that the person him/herself did not know how to deal with this anger. Some children got so angry in response to the voices that they would start a fight outside or at school, or they started screaming at their parents, picking fights with their brothers or starting to hit around with certain things. One boy broke a window with his wrist and another boy chased his brother with a knife.

During the course of the study we noticed that children became increasingly aware that getting angry was a problem. An example: John had regular problems at school as he was getting confused because of the voices and the anger they evoked. A male voice would tell John: 'Just leave it. You never do anything right anyway'. The female voice would then reply that it was not that bad at all. This would then be followed by both starting to argue with each other and very quickly John got confused.

John would get into a lot of fights and he made it difficult for himself. He would look for big, strong boys who he knew beforehand he could never beat. His dad told him that it was this attitude that got him thrown out of the football team. As soon as John entered the dressing room he would start picking fights with his own team-mates. During the study it turned out that John's attitude was linked to the fact that he would overestimate himself and certain situations. He would, for instance, make a mistake at maths by calculating that a cyclist was cycling at a speed of 150 miles per hour. When his teacher asked him whether that was perhaps a bit too fast, to the teacher's surprise John answered convincingly: 'Should be possible ...'. When they did an IQ test, it turned out that John was not clever enough to go to a regular primary school. His inability to understand what was being taught made him feel powerless and he hid that by getting angry. The voices helped him here, John changed schools. This school was far less demanding for him and the problem of overestimating largely disappeared. John calmed down and picked less fights. He formed a drum band and made new friends. In the second year the voices had disappeared.

Alex is another example. During the first interview it became clear that Alex found it difficult to talk about emotions. He preferred to keep himself busy with computer games. Alex's mother was very concerned. She thought that Alex was a highly gifted child and she had organised a number of psychological tests. The teachers at school did not agree with her and the tests did not prove that he was gifted.

Alex started hearing voices for the first time when things were not going well at school and at the same time he learned that his granddad, with whom he felt a strong bond, was seriously ill. He could hardly talk about the problems or emotions that he felt, but the voices could. He felt insecure and the voices made him even more insecure, and Alex could react to that with anger. In the second year Alex changed schools, he started doing well and the voices disappeared. During the third year, the voices sometimes returned, when he felt insecure. He also saw images. According to his mother he had paranormal experiences.

It remained difficult for Alex to show his emotions and, particularly, his anger. Alex found it difficult to get angry and he would try to avoid that, since when he did get angry, things would get out of hand. In the last interview his mother mentioned that last month Alex, in a fit of anger, had hit out at his brother with a kitchen chair. When I asked Alex more details about the fight, I hit the target. He became very enthusiastic and told me that he thought that fights were pretty cool, but at the same time he understood that they were not acceptable. Alex said that his solution to dealing with the anger was to avoid contact with people. He felt most comfortable with that as things could not get out of hand. He would be at his computer and he was good at that. If, for instance, a barbecue had been organised with many of his parents' friends and their children, this was not much fun for Alex. He would withdraw to a little corner where he could be alone. His mother was of the opinion that Alex was a sensitive child who picked up the emotions of others. She was very involved with Alex and, in the meantime, she had followed a paranormal therapist's course through which she could offer Alex support and advice.

It is good to think about your anger, certainly if it often happens that you become unreasonably angry and even more so if the voices make you angry or angrier. You can scare off other people around you. Over time they may not feel involved with you any more, as a result of which you will lose your support. It is better to explain to your parents, friends or your teacher at school what is happening. Whether you should tell your teacher at school depends on the situation. If, during a lesson, you respond to the voices by talking out loud to them, then you almost have to tell your teacher. I have phoned several headteachers in order to explain voice hearing. Most of them were really nice and they cooperated. They wanted to know from me that it was not a disease as such and that you could learn how to deal with it. There are no general rules concerning who you should tell about your voices and who not. It is more a question of whether you can trust the person to help you and I do not mean help you go to a doctor, but help you with your problems at school or at home.

So, if the voices make you angry and you react there are two things you need to do with that. You need to explain things to your parents so that, together with them, you can find a way to deal with it, for example, when you get angry, you briefly go to the hall, or to the loo or at home you can go to your own room. We noticed that parents and teachers did want to listen, but you will have to explain it to them and it is better if you do that when you are not angry. You will come across as more reasonable and therefore it will be easier for them to understand you. Some parents may have had such a shock about you hearing voices that it may take some time for them to get used to it. Please do give them this time, but keep going, don't give up.

The second thing you need to do is think about why you got so angry. What did the voices say or do that made you so angry? What had happened?

TASKS GIVEN BY THE VOICES

Voices regularly give you tasks to do and through this they can have an influence on your life. They can tell you to do things for which you may not necessarily get punished, but that are not nice either. Like Emily, who fancied a glass of hot milk. She warmed up the milk and the moment she looked at the milk in the glass a voice said: 'Throw it away!'

and that is what she did. Emily gave the voices too much power. She did not say 'No, I am not doing that, as I feel like drinking this milk'. In the fourth year she heard the voices less often, but when they were there, she would listen too much to the tasks they set her. Emily had not found a solution for her problem either. She could not handle stress, which made her insecure. She had not finished any school course, had not kept any job. The voices played with her insecurity. Whenever the voices started interfering, she would leave her hairdresser's college or her job as a sales assistant in a shoe shop. The voices would then say: 'Just give up, you cannot do it'.

Laura was told by the voices to only buy black clothes. The examples show that the tasks were not always fun, but they did not cause problems with the people around her. The real problem was that Laura gave too much power or control to the voices. She said: 'I don't even like black'. In the fourth year Lisa still did not have a job, nor a diploma. She was twenty years old, remained at her parents' place and wondered what the future would hold for her. She had no dream about what her life should be.

Problems caused by the tasks set by the voices
You will encounter problems if you listen to the voices when they say: 'Swear at your mum!' or 'Slam the doors!' or 'Break into that car!' or 'Tell you friend he is a queer!' or 'Steal that purse!' or 'You need to steal money, as you need it'. If the voices set you a task during a school lesson and you respond out loud that you do not want to do that, you will run into problems in another way. A teacher does not want you to disturb the lesson.

If you do these things and people do not know that you do them because you are told to do so by the voices, you are seen as an impossible child and you will get a lot of punishment for things you did because you thought you had to. Do not forget that your voices do not share your punishment. You should, therefore, ask yourself whether the things the voices ask you to do are of benefit to you at all? Do the voices have your best interests at heart? If that is not the case, why would you do them?

You have to realize that you will always remain responsible for your own behaviour. If you steal, even if the voices have asked you to do so, you are responsible. Don't forget it is your own hands taking the money.

If you get stuck because you do not dare to refuse the task, you can postpone those tasks that you do not like. You can tell the voice: 'I am going to finish what I am doing now first'. That is regaining control. You can also make a slight change to the task. Jacob was told to kick his little sister and he said to the voices: 'I won't kick my sister, but I will kick a football ten times really hard'.

The voices told Henry to start a little fire. They kept on repeating this task in his head. Henry went to his mum and stayed with her until the voices stopped talking. He could also have asked his mum to light a fire; for example, in the fireplace together.

You can refuse tasks too. Imagine what would happen if we were to tell you to throw a brick through the neighbours' window. Would you do that? Very unlikely. You will always have to keep on asking yourself why you would do what the voices tell you, particularly if it were damaging to you, does not offer a benefit and will lead to you being punished.

OBSESSIVE COMPULSIVE ACTIONS

Compulsive actions go further than being set a task by the voices and obeying them. Compulsive actions are a kind of ritual that you have to perform in order to feel in control of your life. The compulsion to perform the ritual is so strong that you can hardly not do it. Compulsive actions can also happen in children who do not hear voices. If the voices force you to carry out compulsive actions, then there is even more pressure to perform the rituals. Several children in the study told us about compulsive actions. However, it was a subject that they were trying to avoid talking about. They were embarrassed about it.

What kind of compulsive actions are we talking about here? Some of the children had to inspect their room three to five times every night. They were told to look under their bed, check whether their wardrobe was shut and whether the tap in the basin was leaking. When that happens, it takes up a lot of your time before you can go to bed. When Jim was doing his homework in the kitchen, the voices forced him to touch the wall three times or run up the stairs faster than the car passing by his house – an impossible task. Ruth was not allowed to walk on black tiles. Whenever Emily hoovered her room, she was made to do it four times. The voice kept on saying '... again, as it isn't good enough yet'. When you are forced to do these things at home, it is a nuisance, but you can explain it to your family. If you need to make compulsive actions at school, it is a much bigger problem. Children told me that they would think of all sorts of things to make it look natural; for instance, falling over, so that you start doing something again; dropping something on the floor; going to the loo and touching the tiles there.

Compulsive actions do not just happen like that, they are often related to powerlessness; with the idea of not being in control. You can become quite handy at hiding your compulsive actions, but there comes a moment when you will not be able to any more. It starts with the one time when you give in – just walking on black tiles – and the voices seem to think then 'Great, let's set him some more tasks!' At a certain point in time, you will have to tell your parents and they will be disturbed by this. They will probably seek help for you then. It is good if you do not have to be alone with your problem.

An example: because of his compulsive actions Edward asked for help from an alternative therapist and, through this therapist, he joined a group of children that all shared the same problems with their emotions. The therapist asked that they took it in turns in the group to talk about this. When Edward told his story, mumbling as he felt uneasy doing it, she would then say: 'You were going so fast, please do it again'. After that she would say: 'I could not hear you very well, can you tell us once more, but slowly'. In this way, Edward would keep on telling his story about the difficult emotion, until he also felt the emotion and realised it did not kill him. Talking about something regularly helps to calm you down. Research has shown that regularly talking about the voices diminishes the frequency.

Changes

Compulsive actions are pretty stubborn, but we saw changes during our study. The reason that they changed could have been because the rituals were not necessary any more as the problem had changed or disappeared. It could also be that the way the person thought about compulsive actions had changed. In the last interview Edward said about his compulsive actions: 'It is not the voices anymore, but it is me. At the same time I simply do it quickly when I feel it, so I have got rid of it. You see that slice of cake there, I have to eat it and I might as well do that now.'

CAUSING CONFUSION

In the first year more than 50 per cent of the children said that because of the voices they were getting confused. The voices were able to do this by, for instance, making noises, screaming or starting to talk about a different subject than the one the child was occupied with at that time, for example, by commenting on the teacher's dress and saying that it was a stupid dress.

The voices could disturb while the child was doing homework. When a child was busy doing his homework in his room at home, the voices would start talking about things that had nothing to do with that homework, for example, they would start talking about the nice girls at school. That would distract a lot.

The voices could have arguments with each other, which was the case with Josh. The voices disagreed about the advice they gave him. Voices could whisper, which would lead to him trying to hear what the voices were saying and therefore not paying attention to what the teacher said. By talking loudly, the voices were able to mix up the figures in the maths test, resulting in his confusion, which meant that maths, a difficult subject anyway, would become impossible.

It also happened that the voices would make certain work, that the child felt insecure about anyway, impossible. This happened to Megan as the voices would not allow her to do her paper round. She did not obey the voices, but while she was doing her round, they confused her. When she looked at the delivery box, the voices would say: 'You've already delivered there' or 'He has moved' or 'You've already been there'. She started making mistakes which meant she was not doing her paper round well and people started to complain. The voices reacted by saying triumphantly, 'You see, you cannot do it', so Megan gave up her paper round. The voices kept on targeting her insecurity until she gained more self-confidence with the help of a therapist.

If the voices make you confused, this will lead to consequences for your interactions with other people, your social contacts and situations where you need to concentrate, for instance, during school activities. Because of the voices you will sometimes find it hard to concentrate.

How do you deal with getting confused? That is often a matter of making decision. If the voices confuse you when you have to do your homework, you can decide:

1. to do your homework anyway, but to decide how much time it will take you to do your homework; or

2. to decide not do it now, but instead visit a friend and to do it later at night or together with your friend. It is the decision that you make that counts and you have to make this decision with conviction, otherwise it does not work. The voices love it when you are insecure, they like making that even worse.

You can also learn to shut yourself off from the voices. This is a technique used in the area of parapsychology. You can practise this by concentrating very hard on something that you really like, such as a really good book. What you do is to read the words out loud. You only concentrate on the words in the book. You then switch your attention and while you keep on reading, you only listen to the noises around you. As a result you notice that you can decide what you want to concentrate on. You repeat this exercise until you master it.

You can also shut yourself off from the voices by coming to an agreement with them and telling them: 'Not now, but at 7pm'. However you will need to be there at 7pm and give the voices half an hour of your time. You really need to do that then and take the voices seriously, otherwise they remain a nuisance – and angry too. Furthermore, it helps when you can send them away at times that do not suit you, until the moment that you choose to spend time with them.

Changes
The last interview showed that the children who were still hearing voices had learned to concentrate much better. When you concentrate on something, it will be difficult for the voices to get through. You only

have one brain and they need to use it too. If you are using your brain for something else, there will be no space for the voices.

BLACKMAIL

About a third of the children told us that the voices were blackmailing them. Blackmail is really nasty; it can make you completely powerless when the voices threaten to punish you by making too much noise in your head or showing you skeletons, as in Paula's case. They can also threaten that if you do not do what they say, they will kill someone you love or make them ill. For example: Karen heard a voice that said that if she did not listen, her mother would die. The threats were never carried out, but Karen did see a link with other events. Her mother did not die, but she became ill. Karen felt guilty about this disease. It was her fault that her mother was ill. We have seen the things Karen describes happen to other children too. Karen made a link that did not necessarily exist. In her case we have another way of reasoning.

We saw that children who heard voices were often very sensitive. They would pick up emotions or bodily changes in others very quickly. They would recognize these emotions or bodily changes not as if they belonged to the other person, but as if these were their own. So we think that Karen, without realising, picked up changes in her mum. One does not just get ill like that without any signs beforehand. Karen became insecure by what she perceived. The voices love insecurity and they abuse that to gain more power. Karen made an almost mystical link between the voices and her mum's illness. We do not think that it was that mystical, but simply a sensitive child that perceived things very well. In our study we noticed that emotions and voices are not that mystical. Voice hearing is not just limited to the head, but also to the body and all other senses take part too.

Another example: Nadine hears several nasty voices. One voice, her uncle's, can sometimes be nice. He said that on her birthday he would bring her presents. Nadine answered that that would not be possible since her uncle had passed away two years earlier, to which the voice replied that he would be there. The other voices that Nadine heard were nasty since they told her that something would happen to her family if Nadine did not obey them. For example, the voices showed that the whole family were sitting on some dangerous swings. The voices threatened to place the family on these swings so that they would get killed. The threat of her family getting killed was never carried out, but Nadine kept on being scared of the voices.

There is a story behind this blackmail. Nadine's uncle, with whom she had a very good relationship, had committed suicide. As a result of this, Nadine had started hearing voices. She had not got over her uncle's death yet. She could talk to his voice and that is what she did regularly and he would whisper back. It could be that the voices expressed Nadine's fear that the same would happen to her other relatives. It could also be something else. From our studies we are certain that it is linked to Nadine's emotions. Which emotions is something only Nadine can tell us and she does not quite dare that yet.

Nadine's behaviour definitely showed that it was important for her to mourn the loss of her uncle and that her family accepted that she was not ready for it. Her parents were present during the interview and understood Nadine's sadness. Nadine was someone who was hardly able to talk about her emotions. During the course of the study she learned to be better at that. She started to write things down too. In the second year her voices had disappeared. When her grandparents died, she was be able to talk about it. She will never be a chatterbox, as that is not part of her personality.

How do you deal with blackmail?

Voices will start to blackmail you when you give them too much power. They want more and more and even more than that. If you do not set limits, they are very creative in inventing things through which they will get more influence on your life.

How do you deal with blackmail? Our answer is simple and based on own experiences, not with voices, but with real people who can be just as nasty. You have to make decisions. Admit that you are with your back against the wall. Be honest, it can hardly get worse. You have nothing to lose and that is the best position from which to fight back. If you do not break the secret with which they keep a hold over you, they will continue to blackmail you. You have given them a weapon that they will keep on using it. The more you want to keep it a secret, the bigger the power of the voices becomes. If you throw the secret into the open, the situation cannot get worse, but it can get better. This might look like a nice theory that may not be feasible for you right now, but if you want your life back it's something you should start thinking about at some point.

ARE THE VOICES ALWAYS RIGHT?

The stories of the children show that they believe that the voices are always right. We are not so sure about that. How do you know that the voices are always right? When they are talking, it seems as if they know it all, but is that really true? Voices can be wrong too and from what we saw in our study, they were frequently wrong.

You need to have the courage to ask yourself whether your life is going to be controlled by something that may happen or that you dare to take the risk to face up to your problem and start talking about it to someone. You will then notice that things are not that bad after all, that others may have different solutions to your problem and that your fears will never come true. The following proverb applies here: 'Cowards die many times before their deaths'.

Why do you give in to the blackmail of the voices? Because you are embarrassed? Or because you feel responsible for the happiness and welfare of others, but is that right? Aren't you setting yourself an impossible task? The moment you start to think that you are responsible for others, it can sometimes happen that the voices would really like something to happen and, indeed, it happens. If they can make you believe that you are responsible for the life and welfare of others, you are stuck.

Peter told us that the voice threatened that if he disobeyed, his father would have an accident. He ignored the voice and, that same afternoon, his father came home with a lump on his head. He had fallen off his bike. Since Peter started making this link between the voice and the accident, he has turned it into something that could not be solved; as if the voices were completely right and he was responsible for his father´s life. Peter gave in to the blackmail and immediately decided to do what the voices told him to do. It gave him peace of mind, but on the other hand, the voices had a means by which they could control him whenever they wanted. Over time, this could not go on. Peter looked for help and started talking about the voices. He learned that the voices were related to his inability to deal with certain emotions. In the fourth year he did not hear any voices. However, in order to achieve that he had to work hard to change himself. Amongst other things, he had learned to deal with his fear. Peter's mother supported him 100 per cent and that helped him enormously.

With blackmail the same thing applies. It is better to tell someone that you trust and this can be your mum, dad, granddad, granny or your teacher at school. It could also be that a self-help group can help you. Blackmail is something very serious and you need to learn to talk about it, even if the voices do not allow this. Do not keep it to yourself, as that only makes things more difficult. Others can have a totally different view of your problem and they can give advice. It really does not help to withdraw within yourself. It only gives the voices more power.

SUMMARY

The influence of the voices can be very big and can affect your life in a number of different ways. In order to hearten you, the influence changes over time, but you may have to seek help if the influence is too great. We saw that if voice hearers continued waiting passively to see what the voices did with them, they did not learn how to deal with the voices and they would therefore not disappear. So you have to do something about it; try something that suits you. Try to balance the influence of the voices. Try this at home first, try it for yourself first, take small steps and dare to ask the voices questions. Don't become discouraged if they do not answer. One voice hearer solved this problem by telling her voices; 'I will believe in you if you do the washing up for me tonight'. They did not do it and that changed her relationship with the voices. They were not as powerful as they pretended to be.

5

What Happened at the
Start of the Voice Hearing?

In our study we noticed that about 85 per cent of the children started hearing voices as a result of something bad that had happened to them. These bad things could vary, but they always had a lot of emotional impact; for instance, when someone they loved passed away. Some children started hearing voices after having been abused or bullied, but it could also be that the things they were taught at school just did not come across. Children started hearing voices in situations in which they felt powerless and often these were situations for which they blamed themselves; situations in which it seemed that there was no solution for their problem. What did the children in the study tell us about what had happened to them?

CONFRONTATION WITH DEATH

Twenty-three children who started hearing voices did so as a result of the death of someone they had loved or they had dealt with on a daily basis in their lives. We will share a few examples with you here.

Daisy started hearing voices after her granny had passed away. She was 12 years old. Granny had lived next door. Granny's death took the family by surprise and Daisy's parents, aunts and uncles met up in the days before the funeral to mourn together. They did not involve Daisy in this. Her mother said later that they had done this on purpose as they were worried that she would not have coped. It was well meant, but you cannot avoid sadness, you need to experience it, you need to feel it, otherwise it will come out in other ways. It was only after Daisy had been able to talk about it openly, particularly with her mother, that the voices disappeared.

Pete had been occupied with death a great deal since the age of four after his granddad had passed away. He started hearing voices aged seven when Kim, one of his younger brother's classmates, died. It made him very insecure and he would come home crying. Death had had such an impact on him that in the beginning he would take a rose to Kim's mother every single day. Just before Kim's death Pete's family had moved. In this house, Pete would sometimes see the previous occupant walking around. It turned out that this man had hanged himself above the stairs. Things were not going well for Pete. He just could not get on at school. His mum took him to see a psychiatrist, but treatment did not last very long.

When he was about 18 years old, Pete decided to join the marines. During his training, everything was focused on discipline and endurance. He became very strong and self-confident. He was sent to Bosnia. The voices disappeared. He even had the courage to use his vulnerable side by giving a child in his street advice on how to deal with her voices.

Paula started hearing voices when she was eight years old, in the same week that a friend of her brother died. The night before his death the boy had organised a kind of farewell party at Paula's house since he was moving to another city. The boy went home late at night and the next morning they found him dead in bed. The doctor could not find a cause for his death. In such a case, when a death cannot be explained, you cannot just bury the body. The body needed to be examined by a police doctor and that took a while.

Not long after the voices presented, Paula started seeing skeletons carrying their heads under their arms. It scared her a lot. We think that the voices and images showed how she thought about the situation. She could not quite get her head around it. We are saying this as we have noticed that voices often speak in metaphors in order to say something about the problems. If you learn how to translate a metaphor you are probably not that scared of it anymore. However, translating metaphors is not that easy. Paula was helped by a psychiatrist who explained to her that there was a link between the voices and the sudden, unexplained death of the friend of her brother. The voices disappeared in the fourth year.

Mollie started hearing voices after her uncle, a brother of her mother, had committed suicide. He was mentally ill and could not face living any longer. Mollie felt a strong relationship with her uncle. She was an introvert. She could not put her sadness into words, but she wanted her family to recognise her sadness, accept it and pay attention to it.

Sabrina started hearing voices during the funeral of her 18-year-old neighbour who had been her classmate and who had had an accident. Sabrina talked about this: 'His parents were standing outside the church to receive our condolences and I thought: "I will look up at the tree, then I will not have to cry (then I will have everything under control)".' The voice she heard for the first time then said: 'Look at the tree!'

It took some time before Sabrina realised that she finds it difficult to feel emotions and that she prefers to distance herself from them. She concluded that she was in a development phase. Sabrina lived in a village where everyone knew everyone. It was almost impossible to make your own plans, try out what you had thought up yourself and what you felt without others interfering. Sabrina started her degree in a city 100 kilometres away from her village and developed her own identity. The voices disappeared.

After his granddad had passed away, Scott started hearing voices. He was eight years old at the time. Scott had had a good relationship with his granddad. He heard his granddad's voice who invited him to start a fish and chip shop in heaven. Scott was scared of the voice. It was only after his therapist had explained to him that what his granddad had said meant that his granddad did not want to lose him yet, his fear of the voice disappeared and he was able to accept it. During the last year of the study, Jack did not hear any voices any more.

Daisy started hearing voices as a result of her granny's death. The voices disappeared, but they came back when the young conductor of the orchestra in which Daisy was a very active member passed away due to cancer. This time she was not scared of the voices.

John's voices came when he felt powerless and were related to his problem of being unable to cope with his school education. John changed schools, the voices disappeared, but he still found it difficult to talk about his emotions. However, his parents paid more attention to him when emotional things were happening, like the previous year when his six-year-old niece passed away. The whole family were crying at the funeral. John did not, he told his mum he could not. His mum talked to him about this. Both were satisfied with this chat.

Sadness is a very strong emotion, but it could also be that a confrontation with death evokes different emotions than those you had been hiding up until then, like Sabrina who had been shutting out all emotions and, as a result, she had not been able to develop her own 'ego'.

Due to our technical advances, social rituals have more or less disappeared and we have changed death into something technical as it is in a crematorium: music coming out of wall, the push of a button and it is all over within fifteen minutes. Being sad about saying goodbye and crying are taboo; that is for softies. In the past, death and sadness were more a part of daily life. The family or the village became involved. This is still the case in certain cultures. In Ireland, for example, the body is lying in state in the living room and everybody will gather there to pay their respects. People will sit down and have a drink together with the family around the coffin.

The parents of the children who had started hearing voices as a result of death gave these children more attention the next time somebody passed away. This worked.

PROBLEMS IN AND AROUND THE HOUSE

Twenty-three children started hearing voices as a result of problems in and around the house. When the voices start at home, it usually means that you do not feel happy at home. It is a sign that you feel powerless about something and that you cannot see a way out.

Tensions at home
In the case of tensions at home it is not a matter of 'guilt'. Problems at home can be related to the problems of the parents in which the children feel involved, but that they cannot do anything to change. Your dad could lose his job and that would cause a lot of tension. It has nothing to do with you being at fault and it is not your parents' fault either that they are facing problems. People do not really go out and

look for problems, they do not cause these for fun. Talking about being at fault means that you are not getting any further with your problem. You are not looking for a solution, but for someone to blame.

This does not mean to say that parents are never to blame. There are parents who do awful things to their children. This kind of parent did not take part in our study, since people who took part spontaneously replied to our announcement. You would not take part in a study if you abused your child, but you would if you were concerned and you were not sure what was the best thing that you could do for your child.

More everyday parent problems
Paula started hearing voices in the period that her father lost his job. That caused a lot of stress for her mother. She developed severe cardiac symptoms and the doctor feared she might even die. Paula could not cope with her mother's disease. She said that she did not have the patience for this, but we think that she was also scared to lose her mother. Her mother did not know how to deal with Paula's voices. She found them scary and she did not want to have anything to do with them. The voices disappeared when her father found a new job, her mother recovered and everything returned to normal again at home.

Parents with psychiatric problems
Two girls in the study each had a mother suffering from a severe psychiatric illness. These mothers were both very kind and very violent. It is very difficult to live with someone like that. However, and this is even worse, these girls did not learn at home how to deal with emotions. Both girls decided for themselves to take part in the study, since they suffered a great deal from the voices and they wanted to learn more about them.

Sonia heard voices from the day she was born. Her parents divorced and when she was a bit older, Sonia went to live with her dad. Sonia thought that the voices were linked to the unsafe situation (with her mother) in which she grew up. She had started treatment at the mental health centre. Stress factors such as stopping her medication, going to school, falling in love and holding down a job were all emotional situations which had an influence on the voices. Sonia said the following about this: 'My "emotional household" seems to have got confused because of the voices. I cannot feel as I should feel or whenever I feel something a very negative voice appears.'

Abigail had also heard voices for as long as she could remember. Her parents divorced when she was 13 years old and Abigail went to live with her dad. As long as she could remember she heard positive voices, but last year when she had become pregnant by accident and had undergone an abortion the voices turned negative. They had a great deal of influence on Abigail's daily life and she started to think about suicide.

One of the things that Abigail found difficult to cope with was keeping her anger under control. She really lost it sometimes and then became very violent. Therefore she started treatment with a mental health. At the end of the study Abigail had accepted that the voices were her own doing and they represented her emotions. The voices disappeared. She finished her university degree.

Aggressive parents

It could also happen that parents indeed did terrible things to their children, as was the case with David.

David started hearing voices at the age of seven, after he had been hit and locked up in the garden shed for hours. His parents divorced when he was three years old and initially he lived with his mum and her new partner. They abused him. He went to live with his dad, but that did not work out either as he had a full-time job. When he was ten he moved, together with his brother, to a foster family. He started to consider these people as his parents. This foster mother phoned us because of the study. She had consulted a psychiatrist who started to talk about schizophrenia immediately. She did not agree with this label as she blamed his parents for his mental health problems and could therefore not agree with a biological cause.

David heard ten voices of people he knew. These were all people who were involved in the abuse – his mother, her partner, uncles and aunts. These voices had a lot of impact on his life. As a result of what had happened it did not come as a surprise that David had problems with his feelings. If there was tension in his foster family or at school, he got scared or confused. He found anger particularly difficult to deal with.

Siblings being a nuisance

None of the children reported that they had started hearing voices in response to the behaviour of their little brother or sister, but several children indicated that their brothers and sisters had caused problems. Rebecca said: 'One of the things that was linked to my voice hearing was my little sister. I have nothing and she has everything. She is lippy, cool, clever and beautiful.'

We even witnessed that with two boys their 'sweet' little sisters turned into bullies. In both cases the little sisters were socially more adept, they had friends and they behaved impeccably at home. The boys did not have any real friends and their behaviour (part of which was as a reaction to the voices) did not exactly make them very popular either. In both cases I witnessed the little sisters starting bullying and this was not noticed by their parents, but the reactions of the boys to this bullying was noticed even more and they were punished.

An example: John's parents and sister saw me off after the first interview. I had to turn the car in order to drive back and it took a little while before I had managed to turn the car in this narrow street. In the meantime I had a very good view of the family on their doorstep. John stood near his mum and his sister near her dad. I saw the sister bend over and stick her tongue out at John. When he did not react immediately, she did it again. John pushed her. The parents who had only seen the last bit, immediately gave John a clip around the ear. Here a pattern had developed too; John was being blamed, since he was not able to be as sneaky as his little sister.

These may be small incidents, but they do not contribute to a good atmosphere at home. During the course of the study we noticed that both boys developed more self-confidence and they would start to compete with their sisters. They even became more socially adept than their sisters, particularly Ben. He developed into a true 'gentleman'. During the last interview, he took our coffee to the room where we were going to interview him, he opened the door for me and, when we parted, he gave me a bottle of wine as a thank-you present. During the first two interviews things had been completely different. At the second interview, for example, a friend of the parents helped the mother cope with the boy every afternoon. Ben forgot the date he had with me and the friend went out to find him. Ben was punished and sent to his room and I had to go with him if I wanted the interview, so we sat out his punishment together.

However, things can be different too. Brothers and sisters did not have to be a direct cause. Sometimes one child seems to be more happy-go-lucky than the other. One child may breeze through school with great results, is surrounded by many friends and, as a result, triggers unwanted competition and jealousy.

In Ryan's case the voices disappeared when he moved, got his own bedroom and did not have to share with his younger brother any more. The younger brother was good-looking and was able to wind everyone around his little finger. Ryan was more of a Harry Potter look-alike, without the magic tricks. The fact that the voices disappeared when he got his own room must be a sign that he had a problem and felt powerless.

Two sets of twins took part in the study and one of the two would hear voices. These girls had a complicated relationship with their twin sisters where developing their own identity played a role.

Divorce

In six children we saw a link between the divorce of their parents and their voices. Initially the voices would be very supportive and protective, but if other stress was added to this by, for example, changing schools, the voices could turn negative.

Examples

When Joshua's parents divorced, his mum went to live with an aunt. Joshua grew up in an all-female household. After his granddad and uncle had passed away he started hearing voices. Joshua thought that the voices were there to compensate for the loss of his father. He was missing a role model.

Ruth had been hearing voices for as long as she could remember. The year she was born, her parents divorced. She seemed to be able to deal with this pretty well. However, she was scared of losing her mum. When the parents of one of her friends got divorced, it turned into a nightmare for Ruth. Her voices gained more and more influence. For example, when she was tired, a bad voice made sure she would stay awake by telling her stories about her mum getting back with her father.

The voices disappeared when Ruth decided that she wanted to be an adult, go out, start smoking and drinking, wearing different clothes and listening to pop music.

Sonia's parents divorced when she was three and there were lots of fights. Sonia stayed with her mum and, during the holidays, she would be at her father's place. When she was eight years old she started hearing the voice of a fairy who offered her help when she was caught out lying. Since she reacted very strongly to the accusation of this lie, her mother looked for help. The therapist concluded that Sonia had too close a bond with her mum in every sense of the word. During the following years Sonia severed contact with both her mum and her dad. She started to live with a foster family. It was concluded that Sonia had serious problems with setting limits. Sonia was not able to solve conflicts and to develop into her own personality. In the last year of our study she was still hearing voices.

When your parents, both of whom you love, become each other's adversaries and it is silently expected of you to take sides, then something impossible is demanded of you. Your parents are so occupied with their own problems that, in addition, you often feel very lonely. It could also happen that you are concerned that the parent you are going to live with will leave you. Moreover, it could also happen that you feel responsible for preserving your parents' marriage and that you secretly hope that you can bring them together again. Or maybe you feel guilty; you think that the divorce is all your fault.

Sometimes problems keep on piling up. The divorce leads to problems at home and these problems surface at school. School grades get worse. It could be the case that if positive voices are present, these become negative because of the pressure caused by the situation. They can set tasks which could lead to other problems; in short, it is a situation that is making you powerless and you cannot immediately see a way out.

Moving home

Some children started hearing voices as a result of moving house. A two-year-old girl changed completely from the day they moved house. She became incredibly short-tempered. She was sent to a special needs day-care centre and was given medication. Her mother blamed the voice hearing on the move. She got a psychic involved in order to exorcise the bad ghost from the house and that helped a bit.

Gerard's 80-year-old neighbour told him that a farmer had drowned in the well in their garden. The ghost was apparently still floating around in their house and Jerry could have heard him. On the Discovery Channel he had watched a programme which had shown that such a ghost could be present in different forms. Jerry accepted this as an explanation why he had started hearing voices. It worked for him as he was not scared of this explanation.

Mark's voices come and go and they are related to stress. Mark started hearing voices when he was two years old. They disappeared and returned when he was seven and moved. He lost his familiar environment and he was not able to make new friends.

Scott saw World War II images in the attic and heard the voice of a Belgian member of the SS. A psychic explained to him that in a previous life he had been a soldier too, but he had died when he drowned after going through ice. Scott was not particularly enthusiastic about the psychic as such, but his explanation did help.

These examples show that with voice hearing it is not just about facts, or a battle between what is 'true' and what is 'not true' and who determines this. It is about feelings and how best to deal with them.

PROBLEMS AT SCHOOL

Some children started hearing voices as a result of problems at school: bullying by classmates, unreasonable behaviour by teachers or problems related to school performance and abilities. We noticed that, in fact, it could be traced back to hidden problems. Children usually do not talk much about problems at school. Therefore it sometimes took a while before parents became aware of them.

Abuse in terms of bullying, harassment, hitting, kicking and threatening in relation to voices happened reasonably often. Four children had started hearing voices as a result of abuse at school, but there were more children whose voices changed as a result of being bullied. The voices reinforced their anger or insecurity. Almost 40 per cent of the children in the study found that they were bullied more often than their classmates. It could well be that the fact that you are hearing voices makes you vulnerable, even more insecure and, as a result, you are an easier victim of bullying. It is also difficult to divide your attention between your voices and classmates at the same time.

Marina had a twin. The first four years of their lives they lived in a very small village. Marina and her sister spent a lot of time together and they developed their own language. As a result, they were behind in their ability to talk normally. After they had moved and Marina went to nursery school she was not able to talk. At school one of the older children got so mad about this that she banged Marina's head against the wall until Marina reacted by crying. As a result of this abuse Marina started hearing voices. She withdrew even more and it was not until much later that she told her mother.

According to Pauline the voices had started because she was bullied at school. She felt very insecure, was shy and suffered from feelings of inferiority. Pauline started hearing negative voices at school. When she did not pass her grades and had to do the year again, things became easier, the things she had to learn were familiar, she scored better grades and she had much nicer classmates. Pauline enjoyed going to school far more. The negative voice disappeared and instead Pauline heard a positive voice who helped her at school and who supported her when her girlfriends started to criticise her for spending far more time with her boyfriend and not with them.

According to Richard he started hearing voices after he had been bullied badly at school. He was bullied as he was a bit different from the other children and also because of a mild speech impediment (stuttering). He was a loner and very withdrawn. He found it difficult to deal with his emotions. He would get angry really quickly and was not able to deal with his sadness very well.

Several children were bullied at or near school. Peter told us that it would always happen on the school bus, when stronger boys would threaten him. Nobody stood up for him. Pete had red hair and he was bullied about that a lot. Paul had a crooked eye and was bullied about that. The bullying stopped once Paul had undergone surgery to correct his eye. Jack started hearing voices when he changed schools. As a result he had to use a different route and he kept on having to walk past a group of boys who swore at and threatened him. Paula was threatened by three girls. She got so scared that her mother informed the school board. Paula was not the only one threatened by this trio, but she was the only who reacted by hearing voices. The bullying girls were expelled and the voices disappeared.

Unfair treatment by a teacher

Several people told us that abuse of power by a teacher had led to them hearing voices.

Ben's father was in the army and sent to Bosnia. Bosnia was a war zone, therefore there was a chance that he would be shot dead. Ben was completely overcome by emotions about his father's departure, so much so that he avoided talking about it. He did not talk about his father at all any more. At school they noticed his grief, but they did not realise how bad it was. When they did an exercise in class where children had to talk openly about something emotional and Ben tried to talk about his father but could not, his teacher made a fool of him in front of the entire class. His father was home on leave during the summer holidays and that is when Ben started hearing the voice of his teacher telling him to do all sorts of naughty things like stealing the purse of that particular teacher.

Josie had problems and was referred to a psychiatrist. She was embarrassed and did not want other people to know about this. When people hear that you are seeing a psychiatrist they think that you are mad. Unfortunately the only time to make appointments with the psychiatrist was in school hours. When Josie returned to class, her teacher asked out loud, clearly audible to everyone else: 'How was your visit to the psychiatrist?' That teacher had no respect for Josie's privacy. Josie wanted to be swallowed up by the ground. She started hearing negative voices, which made her even more insecure.

Ability problems

Eight children experienced problems at school because of problems related to their ability.

Kasper suffered from several medical problems which made it difficult for him to take part in the normal educational system. He suffered from hearing problems, dyslexia and epilepsy. All these things influenced his school performance. He was not able to keep up. Kasper started hearing voices.

Finn started hearing voices when he was 14. The voices often appeared when he was at school or doing homework and they had a lot of impact then. The voices disappeared when he was 15 which is the age when children have to decide which subjects they will study for their final examinations. After Finn changed subjects and got rid of the most unpleasant ones that he was not very good at, the voices disappeared. Finn also got a different maths teacher with whom he got on much better than the one he had had the year before.

John started hearing voices in the fourth year at primary school when things became more difficult for him at school. The voices were talking about maths and confused him by mixing up all the figures. They also talked about history, geography, art, traffic rules, all the subjects with which he struggled. His parents called on a child psychiatrist but, after a while, they disagreed about the treatment. Neither John, nor his parents, were allowed to talk about the voices. John was diagnosed as schizophrenic and was prescribed medication (Ritalin). They looked for help from a homeopathic doctor who weaned him off the medication prescribed by the psychiatrist and instead prescribed homeopathic medication. John started to sleep better and the voices disappeared. He became less aggressive, picked fewer fights at school and in the street and that is when the real problem became apparent. An IQ test was done and his IQ turned out to be 85. He had insufficient abilities to stay at this school. He switched schools and went to a school for children with learning difficulties. The school switch did him a lot of good. He quickly caught up.

In Joanne's case the opposite happened. She started hearing voices because she was not challenged at primary school. Since she was too clever, she had a special position in her class and she could not cope with that. After she made new friends, the voices disappeared.

Insecurity about own abilities

Changing schools can feel very intimidating: a new environment, new teachers and loss of friends. Some of the youngsters started hearing voices in the first year at primary school when they were around six or seven years old, or during their first year at secondary school around the age of eleven or twelve. When you start something new this always causes a lot of stress and, for some children, it can become just that bit too much at that point in time.

Martin started hearing voices for the first time when he started secondary school, about 18 months ago. Sometimes the voices said that they wanted to help him, but Martin thought that they wanted to make him dependent on them. Furthermore, the voices said that they were strong and powerful. The voices were swearing a lot; for instance that Martin was a fucking pig or that his mother was a slag or a whore.

Pia started hearing voices after she had just started secondary school. In the beginning she did not like her class very much, she felt insecure and she sometimes felt like she was the odd one out. Pia started hearing many voices, 'like a room full of people'. There was a lot of tension at Pia's home. The relationship with her mother was problematic. She started suffering from hyperventilation but, after the voices appeared, this hardly ever happened again. Instead of a physical reaction to her problems, Pia got the voices.

SEXUAL ABUSE, SEXUAL ASSAULT AND RAPE

Sexual abuse, sexual assault and rape are possibly the worst things that can happen to anyone. Moreover, people to whom this has happened are often not believed. So they feel embarrassed and guilty about it, particularly when the abuser is trying to persuade them that it was their fault, as if they have seduced him. If you have such feelings, then you don't dare to talk easily about what has happened to you. Fortunately sexual abuse is less of a taboo now. Several studies have shown that it happens regularly. Amongst the children who took part in our study it had not happened very often, since only children where the abuse had not taken place within the family responded to our appeal to take part in the study. Four children had started hearing voices as a result of sexual abuse.

Katja started hearing voices as a result of a relationship problem that got out of hand. She finished with her boyfriend and classmate Mark, as she had chosen to go out with someone else. The other one was a boy who had contracted AIDS as a result of a blood transfusion. Mark got so angry that, together with a friend, they very aggressively sexually abused her. When she went to report them to the police, she was not able to, since the voice that she had started to hear made her tell a different version of events every time. In order not to get confused she wrote the story down, but then she ran into difficulties with her classmates. They said it was all made up. Consequently, Katja tried to commit suicide.

Ginny was sexually assaulted by a boy who lived next door called Scott. Scott asked two friends to hold Ginny's arms, while he did his business. On the advice of her dad Ginny went to the police. After she had reported Scott to the police, a counsellor advised her to withdraw this. Initially this is indeed what Ginny did, but a few days later she decided to go ahead with it after all. During the second police interview, she started hearing voices, after the policeman who was taking down her story had asked where exactly Sean's hands had touched her and whether she had seduced him or not.

Despite the voices, Ginny stuck to her story. Then her environment started to react to this. Her parents, who had been good friends with Sean's parents up until then, fell out with each other. That became a major problem, since Sean's father was Ginny's father's boss. Ginny's father lost his job. Many other awful things happened in that village and, at the end of the day, Ginny's parents moved out of the village after years of harassment. It was just as bad for Ginny, who had started treatment and who was diagnosed as schizophrenic. After a few years her therapist changed the diagnosis into 'borderline' with the message to the parents that information given by borderline patients can never be trusted. Ginny, whose parents had believed her story of the sexual assault and who had backed her up all the way until then, started to doubt her. Ginny was left out in the cold, since from this different perspective, she could easily have made up the story about the sexual assault.

Laura had been hearing positive voices from the age of six. When she was 12 the voices turned negative. During the course of the following years, she started seeing images and was conscious of another world. Around the age of 15 she began to self-harm. It was only in the second interview of the study that she told us what had happened. When she was 12, her older boyfriend gave her drugs and when she was under the influence of the drugs, he let his friends sexually abuse her. Laura thought that she had provoked this herself and did not dare tell anyone.

Rachel was raped by a friend of her father and started hearing voices. Rachel is from Turkey. She was in an impossible situation. Her father's friend was a regular visitor to her home. Rachel did not dare tell her dad. However, Rachel´s mother offered support and Rachel went to live with her grandma.

These kinds of situation are particularly difficult for girls. Not only do they have to deal with all kinds of very negative feelings like guilt and embarrassment but, when they report it to the police, their environment reacts with denial or anger and certainly not with support. Fortunately, sexual abuse is not regarded as something that people make up anymore. It is accepted as a real fact and recognised as being very devastating. I am not going to deal with it any further here, since enough has been published about it elsewhere.

One more remark. According to the law, sexual assault and rape are crimes and therefore punishable by law. Although the law is very clear, it does not offer any protection from the reactions of other people. It regularly happens that the family prefers to have a 'mad' girl with a psychiatric diagnosis than a father/brother/uncle/granddad in jail. Sexual abuse is a complicated situation where support of people who have been through it themselves can be very important indeed.

LESS FREQUENT CAUSES

Hospital admissions

Being in hospital can be the cause of starting to hear voices, or the cause of the voices turning negative. There were two children who were admitted to a psychiatric hospital whose voices turned negative. In George's case the voices interfered with choices. If, during creativity therapy, he had to choose between two things, the voices would try and make him confused and scared.

Another boy was very often ill and, consequently, in hospital frequently. He was on a ward where it sometimes happened that other children died. He started hearing voices. His nasty voices told him that he was stupid, had to push off, not go to sleep or that he had to do something like scratch himself, hit himself hard or get angry.

Jane was born with a pelvic impairment which meant she had to wear a plaster corset for the first two months of her life. When she was older she started hearing voices, but she still blamed the situation with the plaster corset as the cause of her voice hearing.

Witnessed an accident

There were a few children who started hearing voices during a time of stress and at the same time had witnessed a very severe accident. A girl saw a classmate disappearing under a truck right in front of her own eyes. She did not say a word about this at home. She did not express any emotions about this either. The voices turned very negative as a result of the accident.

Elliot started hearing voices when he was twelve at a time when there was a lot of tension. His parents were building a house and that took a lot longer than expected. In a short period he had to move three times. He also started secondary school at that time and was looking forward to joining his older brother at his school. This did not happen as the teacher of his last year in primary school had made an administrative error with the application for a place at his brother's school. The mistake could not be corrected, since the school was full. Elliot was forced to go to an unfamiliar school. At that time, within the space of six weeks, his granddad and an uncle passed away. Initially he started to sleep badly and hear positive voices. The voices turned negative when he was 15, after he had witnessed a very bad accident. He was standing on a sports pitch close to a friend of his brother who was taking part in a football game on a small pitch near the entrance to the sports complex. This boy was the goalkeeper. During the game, a very difficult slow shot went just past the goal, the keeper tried to get the ball, but he had too much speed and went through a window. The glass severed an artery and it seemed that the goalkeeper would bleed to death there and then. He was as white as a sheet and was hardly conscious. Elliot's mother and brother, who were there too, tried to stem the bleeding, while others called an ambulance. In all this turmoil, Elliot had walked over to the car park and ensured that there would be enough room for the ambulance. The boy was saved just in time. Both Elliot's mother and brother talked about the accident for two days, but Elliot did not say a word. His voices turned negative.

Elliot felt excluded. He was forgotten, despite the fact that he too was close to the accident. During the study's interview we specifically asked about trauma. Elliot denied having experienced something. If someone denies any trauma I explore the past. Elliot and his mother looked back at the time the voices had changed and suddenly Elliot's mum said: '… that was the time of the football accident'. A discussion ensued about what had happened and Elliot told his mum about his role. Now Elliot was able to express his emotions and his mother was finally able to comfort him. She totally understood what he must have felt and she felt stupid that she had not realised it. This was a big relief for Elliot. At the following interview it turned out that the voices had disappeared.

Finding out for the first time that not everybody hears voices

Tanya had been hearing voices for as long as she could remember. She thought that everybody heard voices and when she found out that that was not the case, the voices changed. They became intimidating, a nuisance and negative. There are several children who had the same experience as Tanya. Finding out that you are different can be very daunting. Perhaps it was a coincidence that this discovery coincided with her finding out that she was dyslexic.

Tanya never saw a psychiatrist. Her mother took her to an institute for paranormal experiences and there they labelled her experiences as 'special', but not 'mad'. Hearing voices was a subject that the family talked about openly. Her parents supported her. Later on, Tanya discovered that the voices turned negative at the time when, in a school test, it became clear that she had problems at school because she had dyslexia.

Seeing something scary

Three girls told us that the voices had started after they had seen something scary. One had seen a poster at the GP's surgery with the inside of a child and little men on it; the other as a result of the news around the infamous Belgian Marc Dutroux; another girl told us that her visit to a haunted house had been the trigger for her voice hearing.

Severing a friendship or relationship

Ending a friendship can be very traumatic. Two children started hearing voices as a result of an unfair ending to a friendship. They felt betrayed, deserted and did not know how to deal with that. They could not vent their anger.

Neurological conditions or other influences of a biological nature
The literature shows that there are a number of neurological conditions where patients have described voice hearing or seeing images. These include brain tumours, epilepsy, brain injury caused by trauma, syncopes, migraine, narcolepsy, encephalitis and meningiomas. There are also a number of other symptoms that point to these conditions and voice hearing is for none of these conditions a symptom that is important in establishing a diagnosis. Furthermore, in the literature we can read that blind people were seeing more images and deaf people hearing more voices. In our study various children indicated that they had suffered epileptic fits, but not that these were in any way related to the start of their voice hearing.

The influence of drugs is frequently discussed in the literature, but it is often unclear what kind of correlation there is. There are quite a few voice hearers who start using drugs as a counterbalance to the medication they are prescribed or to escape from the short-term nuisance they are experiencing, but this certainly does not help solve the underlying problems. Some drugs even trigger voice hearing or seeing images. In our study we did not come across children who were using drugs and we did not find any signs of it either. This could well be due to our selection of children.

With six girls their periods had triggered voice hearing. For some, voice hearing had coincided with their first period. It mostly happened in combination with problems at home or school. In the case of others, who were already hearing voices, the voices became more of a nuisance when they were premenstrual. When these girls took Vitamin B at that time of the month, it turned out to work for them. The voices would not get worse then.

Birth trauma
Two boys in our study had suffered a birth trauma. Their parents were of the opinion that this had caused their voice hearing. Both boys had started hearing voices when their development started to fall behind compared with their peers. They became very aggressive and

unmanageable. One of the boys was very conscious about his disability. The thing he wanted most was to get a diploma and that would never happen. Both boys were taking medication to dampen the aggression and, at the same time, they had learned how to talk about their emotions in a better way; amongst other things, about the things that had made them angry.

Brain injury
Jasper started hearing voices as a result of a serious road accident in which he suffered brain injuries.

Anaesthetic
Gregory started hearing voices for the first time when he had a general anaesthetic because he had to undergo surgery. He was scared of death. Gregory started hearing two voices of little metal men.

SUMMARY

In our study, it became evident that in about 85 per cent of the children hearing voices it was linked to one or more traumatic experiences, circumstances or situations. These situations were threatening and the children did not know how to deal with their emotions. These situations reinforced their insecurity and often they felt insufficiently supported. During the research period it became clear that recognising the problem and talking about it helped the children to learn to cope with it and the emotions involved.

6

What Triggers the Voices?

If you want to gain more control over the voices, it is handy to get to know the voices better. What do they do? Are there certain times, situations or activities that trigger or, you could also call it, 'awake' the voices; or do certain emotions lead to the voices becoming active? Children in the study had not often thought of this possibility and therefore not realised that triggers existed. If you do not think about possible triggers, it seems as if the voices come tumbling down out of the blue just like that: as if they have nothing to do with you and only appear to bother you.

In the study we asked at length about the triggers. The majority of children reported several triggers. We started asking about the triggers that were easy to talk about: time, situation and activity.

TRIGGERS

Time

In the first year, 37 per cent of the children indicated that the voices always appeared at a certain time. One of the favourite times was the evening. In the evening you are tired and then you feel less strong. As some children put it: 'That is when I am open to the voices.'

The voices would, for example, appear while they were watching television in the evening or playing cards with their dad. They could appear around the time the children went to bed, or when they were already in bed, but still playing a game or reading a book. Do you recognise that? So how did these children react to the voices?

Some of these children told their parents about the voices and they were given help. For example, the bedroom door would be kept ajar; or parents bought a little night light; or the children were given additional cuddly toys for bed; or their mother would play them soft, calming music; or the mother would lie next to the child in bed until he or she had fallen asleep. In short, parents and child sought a solution together which was feasible for all of them. You cannot demand from your parents that you can sleep in their bed. Their bed is not yours. That might be OK once, but it can quickly turn into a habit that is difficult to break. Moreover, when you receive help because you do not dare to go to sleep, you expect someone else to take on your problem, however that is not how things work. You need to keep on thinking for yourself and trying different things. It is your voices that are disturbing you.

The study showed two things about time: during the years that the study ran, the 'time' trigger seldom changed. It was not as if the voices easily changed the time they appeared. The second point that became clear was that 'time' was a protective factor. In other words, if the voices always appear at the same time, it was easier to learn to deal with them.

Location

We asked: 'Where do you hear the voices?' Locations that were mentioned included: at home, in the street or at school. It became clear that if the voices appeared at a certain location or they became more negative there, it was often that there were problems at these locations. The study showed that just over half of the children always heard voices at the same location, usually at school or in their own bedroom; 20 per cent of the children mentioned that their voices were heard in the same places.

A group of children who mainly heard voices at school had problems at school as they were bullied or not well treated by their teacher, or their academic abilities may not have matched the level of school they were attending, or because they had learning difficulties like dyslexia. We will delve into these problems a bit more deeply, as children often found it difficult to talk to their parents about this.

Being bullied

Of the study's children, 37 per cent found that they were bullied more often than their peers. Lately, fortunately more attention has been paid to this problem openly. Why you are being bullied can have all sorts of reasons. The voices can demand so much attention that it is difficult to pay attention to what the children around you are saying at the same time. That can be a reason to withdraw more and in turn that can be a reason for bullying. A girl was in the same class as three other girls who were bullying her badly. Sometimes she would talk out loud to the voices in class and this was the trigger for even more bullying. At some point the girl told her mother who got so angry that she went to see the headteacher and when he did not do anything about it, she went to the school governors who took some measures. The following year the bullies were not welcome at that school any longer. The girl's voices disappeared during that year at school.

The voices became a problem for an 11-year-old boy when he was bullied in the first year of secondary school about the fact that one his eyes was crooked. The voices would make him angry and in that way the voices helped to deal with the bullying. He had surgery on his eye and the bullying stopped.

Another boy was bullied badly on the bus to school. He could not organise help. A girl's head was banged against a wall by a classmate, because she did not want to talk to this classmate.

Your teacher can treat you really cruelly. An example: A girl called Josie had some problems. She got help and needed to see her psychiatrist during school hours. Josie did not dare talk to the others about this. She noticed that she could skirt around the issue a bit by answering the question where she was going to by saying: '... to see the doctor'. Many people did not enquire any further like: 'What kind of doctor?' and 'Why?' and 'What for?' The answer 'to see the doctor' was enough.

In her new class, Josie had a teacher who did exactly what she had been so worried about. When she returned to class after a treatment session, the teacher would ask out loud: 'So, have you been to see that shrink again?' or 'How did things go at the RIAGG?' (regional institute for mental welfare). At such moments Josie just wanted to be swallowed up by the ground as she was so embarrassed. She suffered from voices regularly in class.

Ben is another example. His father was in the army and was sent to Bosnia, where there was a chance that he could be killed. The thought of that was so difficult for this boy that he lost all emotions. He could not even cry when he went to the airport with his dad. At some point, he tried to talk about this at school, but he could not. His teacher made an instant fool of him. Later he started hearing the voice of the teacher.

The study showed that problems at school can sometimes be solved automatically by going to another school; going to secondary school or with the new school year by getting a new teacher. In these children the voices would disappear as a result of the changes.

Learning abilities that did not match the education level

The first year in primary school presented no real problems for children with leaning difficulties and it seemed they could keep up with their classmates, but after the third year, it became more academically demanding. They felt isolated, the odd one out and that is when the voices appeared or where the positive voices became negative. The children's behaviour changed. They became aggressive. They reacted strongly and picked fights.

John is a good example here. He mostly heard his voices at school. His mother sought the help of a psychiatrist. He was diagnosed with schizophrenia and prescribed drugs. After a while nothing much changed and his mother became dissatisfied. She wanted to get more information and reacted to our advertisement for the study. We interviewed John with his parents present. We were told that his voices had been accepted and were discussed as soon as they caused problems. One of the biggest problems was that John could not stay asleep. He was woken up by a lion with a wild mane and then he would start screaming. The entire family would be woken by it. His mother found a homeopathic doctor who dispensed homeopathic drugs so that he would sleep better. John calmed down. By then he was in the fifth year at primary school and an IQ test was carried out. It turned out he had an IQ of 85 and that was too low for the school he was attending. So John changed schools and the voices disappeared.

Simon had a birth trauma. This was known when he started secondary school. During the first two years at secondary school things went reasonably well but, in the third grade, it became clear that Simon could not cope. He became very aggressive. His parents took him out of school. His father and brother ran a timber factory and he was given a job there. It became clear that he would never be able to function properly. As soon as there was some stress or John became tired, he became aggressive. For Simon, it remained difficult to accept that he did not have a future, as what profession was he supposed to learn? However, Simon did not find the voices negative, as they would help him work out what other people thought of him.

There was also a girl with too high an IQ and that was problematic for her as well. She felt lonely and the odd one out in this world, so she started to make up a world of her own where she did feel at home. She would withdraw into an imaginary flat where she lived with imaginary parents.

Some children had started hearing voices when they moved on from primary to secondary school. They were insecure about their abilities. If you are already feeling insecure and, on top of that, you start hearing voices, you have two problems. This happened to Lillian. She started treatment and was first treated by a psychiatrist who was of the opinion that Lillian should not be talking about her voices. He did not have time for her either during her final exams, when she had asked for more support as the voices had become more active. During her three-year degree course, she had learned to become more assertive and, to the surprise of her mother, Lillian did not want to see this therapist any longer and she demanded to see someone else. Fortunately she got to see a good psychiatrist this time, who explained that the voices were related to her insecurity. She was very satisfied with this. At the last interview she still heard voices, but she was not bothered by them. She had a dream to become an interior designer.

Learning difficulties
You can give it all sorts of fancy names, but the fact remains that dyslexia is a handicap when you are learning. People with dyslexia mix up figures and letters and that does not lead to good grades at school. Saskia was nine years old. She did not do very well at school. She had been hearing positive voices for as long as she could remember, but now that things were not going well the voices had turned negative and Saskia became

scared of them. As a result of the questions asked in the study she started to think about the moment the voices had turned negative. It was at the point when it was discovered she was dyslexic. This in turn had coincided with her discovery that not all children heard voices. She had assumed that it had been perfectly normal and therefore she had never talked about it. Now she felt different.

WHAT HAS COME OUT OF THE STUDY?

Voices often appear at the same location

The study showed that voices kept on coming at the same location. Indeed, it was interesting that if the voices kept on coming at the same location, the chance of them disappearing was greater. This is something you cannot organise, but it seems that when the voices follow more of a set pattern, it is easier for you to learn to deal with them. It also means that there are locations where you feel safe, away from the influence of the voices.

You can think about the question: why do the voices always come at that location? Perhaps you are able to change something about that location or about your feeling there or you can avoid that location. You can even decide a location for the voices yourself; for instance, that you only listen to them when you are in the kitchen. In that way, they will not disturb you any more at the locations where you need to focus your attention on other things like school. In this way, you grant them a location where you do want to talk to them and if they do appear elsewhere, you can tell them: 'Not here, but later on there'.

Activity

About half of the children told us that certain activities can trigger the voices. A few girls told us that going outside was a trigger and that is not such a strange thing when you realise that voices are a reaction to things that you experience which you have no idea how to deal with. These girls had experienced very bad things outside their homes and did not feel safe there anymore. Bad things included being bullied very badly and, even worse, being sexually assaulted. If you do not dare to go outside as you feel unsafe, you are in a situation that is not very easy. What will make you feel safe? Perhaps your mobile phone or your cuddly toy that you can carry around? One of the girls in the study would only go out if her boyfriend came with her and he shared her bed at night. Her boyfriend made her feel safe, but that can only happen if you have a boyfriend.

Another couple of examples: Emily started hearing voices when she was cleaning and hoovering her room. The voices said that she did not do a good enough job. 'Do it again' they would say and they would not just say that once, but throughout the entire morning. Emily had left school as she had encountered difficulties. School caused too much stress for her. She could not find a single school that suited her. She did not want to just be a housewife either. So what else could she do? In the end she decided not to work and to live with her boyfriend and that was the best solution for her.

Paul, who is 15, mentioned that he heard voices during the week. He had been admitted to a psychiatric hospital after a suicide attempt and he was in a ward with peers who often 'let rip of their emotions', as he described it. He could not shut himself off from this and that is when the voices became more troublesome. At the weekend, when he was at home, he did not hear voices. Draw your own conclusion here; is this hospital the best solution for Paul? His father described him as a plant that did not get any water and was withering. In the meantime his parents had accepted Paul's voices and they had also understood that Paul was trying to develop his behaviour in terms of what was good and bad. Paul's parents took him home. The negative voices disappeared and he was left with the voice of a wise man, with whom he communicated every morning and who gave him the strength to live; to walk away from all the bad things of the day.

Philip mentioned that, whenever he was working on the computer at school, the voices would appear. Philip was not very handy with computers and that caused a lot of stress. In Philip's case the voices would appear when he was doing something he enjoyed and then they would ruin the atmosphere, such as when he was drawing. The voices did not want him to feel happy.

In quite a lot of children, the voices would appear while they were doing their homework, particularly when they were doing homework that they found difficult, like maths. The voices would mix up all the figures. Do you recognise that? If your voices appear during certain activities that might be a reason to stop and think here. What do you think of this activity and why?

CHANGES

The study showed that the triggers time, location and activity did not often change themselves, but the problems did change. Problems can change over time, because your life is changing.

With a number of children the voices disappeared during a new school year or when they changed schools. In some cases it was when they started to sleep better and that could be because they were given homeopathic products, or were bullied less, because they had more resistance. It was also important that the children felt they were given more support and that was often at home, but it could also be at school. It happened when voice hearing was no longer a taboo.

SUMMARY

The triggers often changed due to outside influences, as a result of which the children felt somewhat safer and then they learned to develop their own powers and especially their emotions.

7

Voices and Emotions

The voices appear alongside certain emotions, such as when you are scared, sad or angry. That they coincide seems to have to do with the fact you find it difficult to deal with these emotions. You do not dare to truly feel that emotion and you cannot deal with it. When you start hearing voices when you feel certain emotions, they can make you even more scared. That is a real shame, as the reverse is really happening. When the voices start speaking they often tell you where your problem is. However, they happen to do this in a rather clumsy way.

Emotions can be very difficult for various reasons, for instance, because you dare not express them. For example, you cannot feel very sad about something that makes you very sad (and powerless), you cannot even cry about it. You cannot cope with that feeling. Examples are the death of granddad, granny or a friend. It could also happen that things are not going too well in your life and you cannot see a way out, perhaps if you are abused or not wanted. The fact that children can be abused at home is fortunately not denied any more. Not being wanted is a less well-known form of mental abuse. A child can be unwanted if the pregnancy was unwanted, but it could also happen that when a child is a bit older, the parents separate and the father or mother meets a new partner.

These are all things that can happen to you because of external factors for which you are not to blame. This can apply to problems at school too, since the standard at that particular school and the stress this causes was not your choice.

Another reason why you may not be able to deal with certain emotions could be that these emotions bring back certain memories of unpleasant situations that you would rather forget about; something that you are embarrassed about or that makes you feel guilty and powerless. This often happens in the case of sexual abuse or assault, but also with abuse or being unwanted. With sexual abuse it is very easy to say that you (the victim) seduced the person who does this to you (the perpetrator) or by justifying abuse by telling you that you deserved it. We believe that the person who committed these crimes committed another crime by telling you this. A third crime committed by this person is that s/he forbids you to talk to anyone about it, which makes you even more powerless. Furthermore, you could also be blackmailed by the perpetrator by threatening that he will kill you if you open your mouth. As we said before: never let anyone blackmail you, however scared you are. One of the problems with rape and abuse is that you feel embarrassed. Embarrassment is a bad counsellor. The quicker you resolve something, the less damage is done to you at the end of the day. If the person who you are telling what has happened to you does not believe you, go and see someone else, look for someone who you can reasonably trust. Hiding experiences will only make things worse.

Other people could be the reason why you cannot or dare not feel your emotions, but it could also be caused by something within you. It could be that you have a reason why you have never learned how to deal with a particular emotion. For example, you may have decided that you will not allow yourself to get angry, because you have noticed that when you get angry, you cannot control yourself and you are scared to lash out and hurt someone, or you may think that you cannot fend for yourself. If you really believe that, you are stuck. You could say that voices are a reaction to something that is (still) a problem for you.

FEAR

Most children were scared of the voices when they experienced them for the first time; scared of what they said, their threats, the memories they brought back; scared of the voices because they were making accusations or were critical of things the children felt insecure about anyway.

Many children also told us that fear was a trigger in itself (67 per cent). So when they were scared, certain voices would appear. There are quite a few things of which you can be scared; the dark, certain movies or certain people in your environment. Do you recognise any of these or does something else scare you? Are you scared already and do the voices scare you even more. You are so scared, in fact, that you feel as if you are paralysed. This happened to 15 per cent of the children. The voices would scare them so much that some children did not dare to listen to what they said (12 per cent).

An example of fear aggravated by a voice: Paula lived in a narrow street. Her grandfather's house, which was right opposite Paula's, was burgled. Of course, everybody at Paula's place talked about this a lot. They were trying to imagine what it would be like if a burglar were to come to their house. It really scared Paula and her voice loved that. He explained in detail how the burglars had got in. As a result of his story, Paula saw a potential burglar in every stranger she walked past in the street. Therefore, she spent a lot of time watching to see if there were any burglars in the street or not. It made her suspicious and even more scared.

Your fear can become less if you do something about it yourself, but it could also be that others need to help you with that. We noticed that it did not really work if parents tried to prevent fear. It simply did not work. You can hardly lock your child in a little box and not let it move any more. Moreover, it would probably get scared of something else then – that there would not be enough air or food, etc. No, you have to face it. In real life there are things that will scare you, so you better learn a way to cope with it.

Fear is part of daily life. If you get scared often, you should start wondering whether it is real or whether your fear is exaggerated. For example, fear can help you move safely through traffic. Fear should not be so strong that, out of fear of an accident, you do not dare to cycle any more. That is when you give fear too much room to play.

In our study some parents told us that when their child was scared at night, they would let the child into their bed, which meant the fear became a family problem over time. The parents could not sleep well, because of having an unsettled child in between them. That was not good for their mood. And on top of that, one cannot really afford to be sleepy at work during the day. We also know some parents who, when things got too much, learned to say to their child: 'All well and good, but you sort it out with your voices, it's nothing to do with me', when, for instance, the voices started to interfere with the choice of clothes or the habits of the parents, like the voices who made it impossible for the parents to go out or do something on their own or voices that forbid a certain colour in the house.

Changes

During the first year of the study the fear changed in more than half of the children. They learned how to deal with their voices and therefore they were less scared. They would not let the voices scare them so much any more. The example of Laura: 'I have become more critical towards the voice and I have started to check whether the things the voice claimed were true. Often that was not the case. I am less scared of the voice now.'

It could also be that the problem changed, as was the case with Jacob. He encountered problems at school and changed schools, where things went well for him. He felt more appreciated and stronger. Not only did the voices appear less often, but also his relationship with the voices changed. They became more positive and started to give him advice.

Summarising

Fear is a positive emotion as such. Fear protects you, warns you of danger. For example, you should not cross the road without looking first. On the other hand, not everything is as dangerous as you might think. If you avoid learning to deal with your fear, your world will become very small, like the two girls in our study who were scared to go outside alone. They only dared to venture outside if their boyfriend, parent or someone else came with them.

ANGER

Anger is another important emotion and, for some children, a difficult emotion that they cannot deal with. Anger is a very normal emotion, but if it is caused by abuse or by someone who makes you powerless, it becomes a very difficult emotion. You are not able to hold your own against the person who abuses or sexually assaults you and that makes you incredibly angry.

Fortunately anger is very rarely for these reasons. It is far more common that children cope badly with the often normal arguments with other family members. They do not know how to manage their anger at all. It is also very common that children are not taught how to handle anger as, in many families, it is thought that anger is a very unpleasant emotion. If that is the case, it is very difficult to learn to deal with it.

Anger can also be a logical result of being bullied. It often happens to children who cannot speak up for themselves very well and, therefore, they do not know how to deal with their anger either. If anger is a problem for you, you need to think hard about why it is a problem and you may need to find someone to discuss this with.

Many children told us that anger had been their trigger for the voices (52 per cent). There are different ways in which this trigger works. If you are angry, the voices will appear and aggravate things. You get so angry that you become a problem for the people around you.

An example: A boy was being bullied by his brother and could not express his anger. He got hold of a knife and chased his brother around the house. His mother was totally shocked by this. There is another way too. For example, you are angry with your dad or your brother, but you will not allow yourself to express it. Instead of the anger, the voice appears.

Ben cannot manage his anger. He does not allow himself to get angry and reacts very strongly to anger. When he witnessed fights in the streets the whole background became a blur and suddenly this figure appeared like a referee in between the people who were fighting. He felt responsible for all arguments. Ben: 'When I see an argument, I think, "I will come between them …"'. At night, after such an argument Ben would see shadows in his head and he heard the voices of monsters.

So, anger is a problem for many children. Learning how to deal with it is not a subject they teach you at school. You need to learn it yourself. Anger, often referred to as aggression, is, in fact, taboo in our society. We are scared of anger. Aggression is allowed as long as certain rules are set first, like in sports, for example, in a boxing match. The whistle is blown on those would do not stick to the rules. (However, with football something strange appears to happen. Although the players have to stick to strict rules and get punished at the slightest show of violence, the supporters often display very aggressive behaviour. This is socially unacceptable but, even so, it is a fact. So far no solution has been found for this problem.)

If you do not know how to handle your anger, you can also react by completely clamming up. You probably feel that your power was taken away from you. Powerlessness is a very negative emotion.

Alex, for example. During our third encounter it became very apparent that talking about emotions still did not come easily to Alex. He tried to avoid my questions with all kinds of little tricks. 'Yes' and 'No' were perfectly good answers according to him. Changing the subject was another of his strategies. However, in the end he wanted to cooperate. He admitted that he could not get angry very easily. That was his biggest problem. He said that after his mother had mentioned this last month, Alex, in a fit of anger, tried to hit his older brother with a kitchen chair. When I asked Alex for more details about this fight I hit the bull's-eye! After that, he was prepared to talk more about his emotions. Alex's solution to handling his anger was to avoid contact with people. He preferred working on his computer. If, for example, his parents organised a barbecue with many friends and their children, this was not exactly fun for Alex. He would find a little corner where he could be alone. His mother offered another explanation. She thought that Alex picked up other people's emotions and he was completely lost about what to do with them. That is why he preferred to be alone. Her explanation allowed her to accept Alex' behaviour and support him.

Alex may still have an anger management problem, however, quite a lot has changed during the course of the study. He has clearly gained more self-confidence. He has a girlfriend now and things are going well at school. He gets angry less often. Everybody has their own speed at learning how to deal with problems and so has Alex.

Perhaps you need to stop and think how you can deal with anger in a different way than letting it explode or locking yourself up within yourself. Perhaps you need to learn to recognise your anger earlier and start talking about it when you can still behave in a reasonable way; perhaps you need to learn first how to express your anger in a different way – by hitting a pillow, enrolling in a boxing class or learning how to play the drums. You also need to realise that extreme anger or isolating yourself can alienate you from other people which means you could make enemies. Will that help? Is that your aim?

Changes

During the course of the study anger changed in quite a few of the children. They learned how to deal with it in a different way; they would not allow the voices to make them so angry. Some children learned, almost accidentally, the things they experienced in life. Though a few children made a conscious decision to learn how to do it. They enrolled in a course which taught them how to behave assertively, or a boxing course or judo. They learned to recognise their own power and how to stand up for themselves more. In that phase of your life, the only thing that is feasible is recognising your problem and indirectly you learn how to deal with this emotion.

SADNESS

In almost half of all the children (49 per cent) the voices would appear when they were sad. Sadness is another difficult emotion that you are not supposed to show in our society. Here we are taught not to cry. That is childish, you are a softy if you cry. If you are sad and you cannot do anything with that emotion, you can become depressed. Our society likes depressed people even less.

About 21 per cent of the children told us that the voices had appeared for the first time after someone they loved had passed away. Daisy started hearing voices when she was 12 after her grandmother had died; her mother's mother who had lived next door. Initially she heard a voice, then she heard three voices and sometimes a large number of voices. In 1993, when we organised the first conference for children hearing voices, she was supposed to give a talk in which she would talk about the voices and the death of her grandmother. We had practised her talk at least three times and she never struggled. On the day of the conference, Daisy spontaneously burst into tears during her talk. Her mother who was sitting in the front row was completely shocked. Afterwards Daisy was able to talk to her mother about her grief as a result of her granny's death for the first time. It was not as if her mother had not wanted to listen to her; on the contrary, she had not wanted to discuss death as she was concerned that Daisy could not handle it. Not long after the voices faded away.

The voices returned when Daisy was once again confronted with death. The young director of the orchestra in which she was a very active member died of cancer. His death made her very sad. However, she does describe that she was able to grieve. There was a memorial service where everybody cried. This time she was not completely taken by surprise by the voices and she was less scared of them.

How do you learn to deal with death when you are that young? Most adults are scared of death. Just look at the literature and movies. Adults prefer to deny it and offer a reasonable solution. Life after death makes death less absolute. That is all well and good, but the fact remains that when someone dies you will never see them again. Their body disappears. That is very difficult to accept, as not only will you never see the person you love any more, but at the same time a piece of yourself also dies, since no new memories are created and the old ones fade with time.

Changes

During the course of the study, the attitude towards grief and sadness only changed in a handful of children. It remains very difficult to deal with grief and sadness, even more if you don't know how to express it, by crying for instance.

For example, John. John still finds it difficult to deal with his emotions, let alone talk about them. His parents pay more attention to him at emotionally difficult moments like recently during the funeral of his little niece who was only six years old. Everybody cried. John could not, but this time at least he was able to tell his mother that he could not cry. His mother dug deeper into this and they had chat about death and grief. No voices appeared for him at this time.

FEELING INSECURE

There are quite a few children who feel very insecure and doubt their own opinions – the voices love that. They jump at the chance (37 per cent). For example, when Pia feels insecure the voices say: 'You simply cannot do it' and that makes her feel even more insecure. Several children hear this. Their own self-doubt is put into words by the voice. Insecurity or self-doubt can be related to school performance or in sports, and also to making choices. A few children, for example, had started hearing voices after they had changed schools.

The voices hardly ever agree with Millie's choices. For example, when Millie needs to choose between a pink or blue bottle of shampoo she will choose the pink one as she is a girl. The voices make her insecure by telling her to take the blue one. In order to keep them happy she obliges.

If you let the voices choose, they can go too far, like the girl whose voices started to decide everything, from what she was going to have in her sandwich to what to wear and what to eat in the evening. The funny thing is that you allow the voices to take that much power. Being given advice can be a good thing, but if you start to eat things you do not like, you have given the voices too much power. Imagine if your parents or boyfriend were telling you to eat something you didn't like. Would you do that?

Changes

Millie was by far not the only one who felt insecure when she had to choose. We noticed that, as they got older that the children learned to make better decisions themselves, as opposed to following the choices of the voices. Some had invented a system for this. If they had to choose between two things, they would award both a score. They would choose the one with the highest score. Or they would imagine a pair of scales and on each side they would place one of the things from which they had to choose. They would choose whatever made scales tip to one side, or they would look at the price. They would choose the cheapest.

In the fourth year, quite a few of the children told us that they had far less trouble when having to make a choice. Floris said the following about this: 'Last year I still found it difficult to choose, but that has changed now. I don't find that difficult any more, as I know what I want now. To give an example: in a restaurant if I have to make a decision about what to eat, then I will choose a dish that comes with chips as I like chips.'

The study showed that children who had become patients kept on having problems with feeling secure. We saw that often other people make the decisions for these children.

FEELING GUILTY

Guilt feelings are very difficult as they are often linked to feeling embarrassed or ashamed and you'd rather not talk about it. Therefore it is often an emotion that you keep to yourself and people around you don't know anything about it. If you don't talk about it to anyone, you can dwell on it and it could perhaps be that your thinking is wrong.

Particularly in a situation where you feel powerless, guilt feelings often crop up. When you are abused, you immediately think that it is your fault. Even if you did not think of this yourself, the person who abused you will tell you that it is your fault. Your behaviour triggered his behaviour. An unpleasant example is a priest who sexually abuses a young boy and subsequently tells the boy that it is his own fault as he seduced him. Never let people make you believe that when they lock you up in a shed, abuse you in whichever way or sexually abuse you, that it is your own fault as you lured them into doing this.

It can also happen that you think that you are responsible for the happiness of your parents' marriage. If they get divorced it is your fault. Don't do that to yourself. Divorce is a complicated issue concerning the two adults who married. As a child you are the victim in the divorce and not the one who is responsible. If you cannot talk about those kinds of feelings, the voices will do that for you and mostly not in a helpful way.

Changes
During the course of the study the trigger 'guilt feeling' disappeared in the group of children who had not needed therapy. This did not happen amongst the children who had become patients – they kept on feeling guilty. Guilt feelings can be very stubborn. If you keep on feeling guilty, you are not able to let go of the past and focus on the present. That is

easier said than done, but not letting the past play a dominant role in the present is possible, particularly by having the courage to talk to others about your guilt feelings. However, the problem you feel guilty about needs to stay in the past. Talking with someone you trust is necessary too, and if that is not possible with 'Childline' for instance.

BEING ALONE

Not everybody likes being alone. A number of children start hearing voices when they are alone (32 per cent). If you are alone and not doing anything, you are open to voices. You are not being distracted and the voices can keep you pretty occupied. This can happen in a positive way too. For example, we know someone who is very much alone and he agrees to meet the voices in a cafe in order to have someone to talk to when having a coffee. This man does not want to get rid of his voices at all, but he is not involved with his voices all day. He makes sure that he has lots going on in his life.

It could well be that if you spend a lot of time on your own – and that can happen if things are not going too well for you anyway, or if you are in hospital, for example, that the voices will want your attention too often and for too long and that is not a good thing. There is more to life than voices.

It is difficult to find distractions when the voices scare you a lot, confuse you or when they have too much influence on the way you deal with the world around you. For some children a set daily pattern was a tool to keep them from being alone too much and therefore to not being too occupied with the voices. You can also try to give them your attention at a set time each day and then clearly tell them at all other times: 'Not now, but later'.

FEELING UNHAPPY, HAPPY OR BEING IN LOVE

The voices enjoyed reinforcing certain emotions and that particularly applies to feeling unhappy (17 per cent), feeling happy (12 per cent) and being in love (8 per cent). As with all emotions voices can reinforce your feeling in a positive or negative way.

TALKING ABOUT YOUR FEELINGS

It is very important for all children and adults who hear voices to learn to talk about their feelings, even if these are difficult feelings, that one is ashamed of and doesn't know how to deal with.

If you do not learn to do that, the voices will talk about them, but if you learn to talk about these feelings you can develop further until you do not need the voices any more, or the voices will change from being intimidating to being your support. Since it is so important to talk about them, I will give you an example below.

Example – Ben

Ben discovered that he was very strong and he thought that if he got angry he would truly knock someone out. As a result, he got scared of getting angry. He decided not to get angry any more. Through this reasoning he made himself powerless. The voices started to interfere. At the slightest thing the voices would get angry and that made Ben very angry. Sometimes the voices caused Ben to make others angry; for example, by confusing him when he had to write down his homework. When he got home afterwards, he had no idea what kind of homework he had to do and it drove his mother mad.

Ben was set all kinds of tasks by the voices, which caused him problems too; tasks which made him late for school or getting home. He was told to jump off the roof (something he did not do) and start fires (something he did do). In short his parents found him unmanageable. He, on the other hand, thought that his parents were setting too many rules. He considered that he was punished too often.

During our fourth encounter, Ben told us that he had learned to deal with his emotions, particularly his anger, in another way. He learned how to deal with it with the help of his teacher at school. If, at school, he felt powerless because of his anger, he would go up and talk to his teacher. The teacher would then ask the boy with whom Ben had the argument and was angry to come and talk to Ben in order to solve the problem together. That worked well. The key problem was that Ben had always thought that he was responsible for all arguments. He thought differently now. He said: 'Getting angry once and having an argument is possible, but if this happens frequently about the same subject, then it's not my fault, but someone else's.' Since he began to think about it this way, he felt freer. So Ben was still getting angry, but he didn't let it get out of hand any more.

Ben was not as scared when he was out as he used to when he would often think that he was being followed. He even enjoyed being prewarned by the voices about some boys hanging around at the corner waiting to beat him up. He still had a lot of self-doubt, but he said the following about this: 'That is part of me, I will always be like that'. During the last year, Ben did not hear any voices. By now he had an inner dialogue. In case of problems, he would tell himself: 'Just sit down now, don't say anything, in this way you won't encounter any problems'.

SUMMARY

Voices have everything to do with emotions, particularly those emotions with which you have difficulty dealing with. However, you can learn how to deal with them. During the period our study ran we taught all the children in the study to deal with their emotions in a better way. Some learned by choosing to enrol in a course or some classes, others by seeing therapists and others learned this by being open to the advice of others. Life will teach you, but you have to be open to it.

8

What Explanations Are There for Voice Hearing?

Usually, when you do not understand something, you try to find an explanation. Through this explanation you think you understand it, give it a place and it becomes less scary. Furthermore, an explanation helps you to talk about it with other people. You can exchange experiences and you do not feel so lonely or different.

When you start hearing voices, most often you do not know what is happening to you and you do not have a language to talk about it. At that point it is necessary to get a language and explanation so that voice hearing will start to fit into your life. It will become part of you and you learn to accept it. That sounds nice, but what do you do next?

The explanation you have found for your experiences determines the way in which you deal with them. If you think it is a disease you need to go and see a doctor who can help cure you. If you think that it is normal in itself, then you need to learn to deal with it, but that means that you need to find out for yourself what suits you and you usually learn more doing it that way, rather than leaving it to someone else.

Our study showed that adults spend a lot of time looking for an explanation. They hit the library and start reading. This did not happen so much amongst the children in our study. I think that it may have to do with the fact that their parents were pretty occupied with this and when someone else is doing it for you, you do not feel that much of a need to do it yourself. Most children thought that voice hearing was a paranormal gift. Most of them did not quite know what that meant; it was a term they had learned from their parents. According to them, paranormal had something to do with predicting the future and with another, non-material world. However it mostly had to do with receiving help and advice. It sounds positive and interesting when you have this paranormal gift; you can tell your friends about it, but it can be quite scary too. If the voices tell you that your father will be involved in an accident, you will get scared. It could be that you start to feel responsible for the welfare of your father. It could happen that if the voice tells you that someone has a very serious disease, you do not dare to look that person in the eye anymore. What are you going to do with the information that you are receiving via your paranormal gift?

I think that it may be a good thing to find out first how much of a gift you have and whether you feel the desire to do something with it. Not everyone has this desire.

There are only a few children who are hugely gifted in this way. A boy in our study was immensely gifted and, at the young age of 16, he was able to give others advice about their health. He was guided by an aunt who had this gift too. It was quite a learning curve. I know of another child who was advised to wait a little longer, since he was still too young. Several children went to see a paranormal healer and these people taught them how to deal with their experiences. If you believe that your voices are a paranormal gift, this is a positive explanation as such, which does not make you powerless.

Children who told us that their voices came from another world, or were ghosts or phantoms, also used explanations that were socially accepted. You only have to look at the literature. Many books have been written about extraterrestrial beings and about phantoms. Phantoms and ghosts can make you scared, but you can do something about that. In most books they are fought off and conquered. You can ask your parents to help you. There was a girl with an Indonesian mother and, for her, the explanation of ghosts from another world fitted with her mother's culture.

THE POWER OF EXPLANATIONS

There are explanations that keep the power with you. We mainly saw that in the older children who, during the course of the study, had become convinced that the voices had to do with themselves. 'I now think that it is me,' Pia says, 'but there are two sides to the coin. On the one hand it is comforting that it is me, but on the other hand, it makes it more difficult too. Do I have to do something about this myself?' According to Tilly: 'I think that the voices are caused by too much stress.' Monique says: 'I think that the voices have to do with me; with my way of dealing or not dealing with emotions.' In Cathy's case the voices function like a conscience, because of her guilt feelings.

There are explanations that make you powerless. Half of the children went to see a counsellor. There, they were confronted with the opinions, theories and language of the counsellor. According to Alice, voice hearing is a disease and she is crazy. Her answer to the question, why she hears voices is: '... because I am sad or crazy'.

Alice was sexually assaulted and, as a result of that, she started hearing voices. Her explanation that it is a disease leaves her powerless. She was diagnosed as schizophrenic which was later changed to borderline and, to be honest, that did not really help her an awful lot. On the contrary, she lost the support of her parents as the psychiatrist who gave her the diagnosis of borderline explained to her parents that borderliners often lie.

EXPLANATIONS, PARENTS AND SUPPORT

Earlier I was talking about you, the voice hearer. In this part I would like to explain something about your parents, as you need their support.

It is pretty difficult for parents to cope when their child starts to hear voices. They see their child's fear and pain and they want to do something about that. They look for help, but from whom? That is where finding an explanation pops up again. If you think that it is a disease, you will go and see a doctor. Unfortunately the disease model is based on the fact that the voices are a delusion that you should not talk about. Most parents of the children in the study were scared of psychiatry or had had bad experiences of it. Usually quite a lot had to happen before these parents dared to find their own way. It is difficult to tell a doctor that you believe that he has got it wrong. For example, a psychiatrist told a boy who heard voices: 'First you get scared and then you make up these voices'. The boy disagreed. It was the other way around. He first heard voices and the voices scared him. His parents supported him and stopped his treatment.

Mothers seemed more prepared to accept their child's explanation and to support and fight for them than fathers. Several mothers asked me to phone the teacher or headmaster in order to explain that their child was not crazy and that voice hearing is prevalent in six per cent of the normal population.

Mothers also supported their children within the family. Let me give you an example here. During our first interview Eric had a physical reaction when he spoke about the voices. He turned pale and sweated. He could not find the right words for this experience either. Eric's mother told the female interviewer that her child was sensitive and had a gift. 'Nonsense!' said the father who walked in at that point. 'He is just clumsy. He can hardly cycle.' Fortunately for Eric, his father's explanation was not decisive. Eric's mother found that he needed help, but her GP knew practically nothing about voice hearing and she did not want to go and see a psychiatrist. During the second year Eric, together with his mum, went to see an alternative therapist. In meetings with other children Eric learned to talk about his experiences. During the second interview he had no physical reactions any more and could talk quite clearly about what he experienced. During the study Eric and his mum regularly attended meetings organised by the therapist where he could talk to fellow sufferers.

SUMMARY

Being able to talk about the voices is important, but in order for this to happen they need to have been accepted. Unfortunately there is not just one explanation. That would be easy. There are many explanations for voice hearing. The explanation you give for your voices determines the way you deal with them. There are explanations that make you powerless and there are explanations that give hope stimulate you to find your own way with the voices.

PART 2
The Stories of Eight Young People

Why Did We Choose These Stories?

In this part you will find eight stories of children who hear voices. They all took part in the study. Two of the children we had met three years before the beginning of the research when we organised the first congress at Artis Zoo in Amsterdam for children who hear voices. The actual research finished in 2002, but we have kept in touch with several of the children. So we have known the children/youngsters for a while. Their stories show what it is like to hear voices and how it can affect you.

Pete had been hearing voices from the age of four after he had been confronted with death. Up until his adolescence the voices were a real pain. His education did not go well and he simply did not know what to do with himself. He decided to become more active and entered into a different relationship with the voices after he made the decision to apply for a job as a marine. The very tough training gave him the physical power he needed to learn to set limits to the voices. Throughout his entire story, his mum's support is evident. She accepted his experiences and, together with Pete, she looked for a way in which to deal with this in his life. He learned to talk about it. The voices disappeared but, by now, he has an internal dialogue.

Paula started hearing voices and seeing images when she was nine, after the death of her brother's friend. It made her feel very insecure. The voices were overwhelming and that scared her a lot. Her mother could not accept the voices, but she did fight for Paula at school when she was bullied. Paula's father accepted the voices and supported her at home. Furthermore, Paula was given the help of a psychiatrist who explained to her that the voices were probably linked to the death of her brother's friend. Paula's voices would also change when the situation changed; for example, when problems at school were getting worse. Once Paula learned to deal with her emotions in a better way and she met a new friend with whom she could talk about the voices and changed schools (from primary to secondary), her voices disappeared.

John started hearing voices when he was nine, when things were not going too well at school. John could not talk about it or deal with it and started picking fights. When his parents looked for psychiatric help, the psychiatrist talked about him being schizophrenic, prescribed medication and did not allow him to talk about the voices. Both parents were dissatisfied with the treatment and therefore decided to take part in our study. They asked us whether we knew another therapist. We knew a homeopathic GP who worked with children hearing voices. This man prescribed homeopathic drugs which helped John to become less angry. Following that, the entire problem came to the surface. John's IQ was 85 and, because of this, his school was too difficult for him. John changed schools and the voices disappeared. After that, John was still not able to talk about his problem, however much his mother tried to encourage him. He was not able to deny that he had a problem, but he could not feel any emotions about it. In the fourth year of the study he started hearing a voice again, but the voice just flashed past and did not say proper words. John did not find that voice interesting at all. There was more to his life now – like his drum band.

David started hearing voices when he was seven as a result of serious abuse by his mother and stepfather. He was placed with a foster family where his foster mum supported him all the way. This was sometimes tricky, as David's voices were putting her down all the time. The voices set tasks, were nasty and caused a lot of nuisance for David and because of David's behaviour towards those around him too. When his foster mum went to look for help, twice she encountered therapists who started talking about schizophrenia. She did not go back to them. In desperation, her GP referred her to a hospital where the voices were accepted and not considered an indication of disease. David's problems were not denied either – abuse from your mum is something you will never forget for the rest of your life.

David was advised to go to boarding school. He discovered that he was a very talented cyclist and he went to a boarding school for cyclists in Belgium. It was there that David developed into a strong athlete and, according to him, it helped him set limits on the voices. Two years later I had telephone contact with David's foster mother and she said that he was doing well and the voices had disappeared.

Emily started hearing voices when she was seven. Emily had always been a very obedient child, but now she started to do all the things the voice told her to do. She started suffering from obsessive compulsive behaviour and left school. After a short admission in a psychiatric hospital, Emily decided that this would never happen again. She started another school; it did not work. She tried another one and that did not work out either. Every time Emily suffered from stress or had to perform, the voices would make it impossible by confusing her or by setting her tasks. Emily received a lot of support from her mum and her younger sister.

In the fourth year, Emily gave up hope of ever having a profession. She was sitting at home alone waiting for the house she had bought with her boyfriend to be ready. She still hears voices, but they were pleasant, since she was less alone then. The voices still had some control over Emily and she was OK with that. There were no family conflicts, not with the voices. It was her choice and her life, but in doing so she hampered her development.

Ben started hearing voices and seeing images when he was six. Ben's voices changed with his mood. His voices forced him into all kinds of behaviour that got him into trouble. His parents did not know what to do with him at all, but they did not want to go and see a psychiatrist.

As a consequence of Ben's behaviour it was difficult to understand his real problem – that he could not manage his anger. He reasoned that, if he got angry, he was so strong that he would beat up the other person. A teacher at school taught him that being angry with someone did not mean smashing them to pieces, but that you had to talk to the other person. You needed to explain why you were angry and understand why the other person was angry. After Ben understood this, he changed. He became a nice person to live with at home, got new friends and became popular at school. His voices disappeared. He has an inner dialogue now.

When Laura was six years old she started hearing voices after her grandma died. By the time she was eleven her voices had turned negative. Later she would harm herself. At eighteen she was admitted to hospital; there were too many conflicts at home. Laura was prescribed medication and saw both a psychiatrist and a psychologist, but never told them what she told me. When she was eleven her boyfriend, who was 23, had given her weed and subsequently sent his friends to her bed. Laura had experienced gang rape and felt like a whore.

Laura was diagnosed as schizophrenic and prescribed medication suitable for this diagnosis. Laura dissociated (lost time) a great deal, but no attention was paid to this, although it is a clear sign of trauma.

When the hospital closed Laura went to live at home again. Rules were set and she was given a horse and started a part-time job at a riding school. This structure in her life helped her deal with the voices. She became more independent.

Despite the fact that Laura's mum supported her, gave her a lift to work, and would ride with Laura, she only saw Laura as an ill person. She was offered a course on how to deal with a schizophrenic child, but Laura never told her mother what had happened to her. Laura's secret continues to make her vulnerable.

Daisy started hearing voices after the death of her granny, when she was not involved in the grieving process. The voices disappeared after Daisy had been able to openly cry about this loss.

Daisy's voices were a mirror of her well-being. They returned when she was confronted with difficult emotions, such as a repeated confrontation with death. Despite the fact that Daisy was very independent, she did not make things easy for herself when she was one of two girls enrolling on a civil engineering course. She accepted the reactions of the voices and she found a reasonable balance in her dealings with the voices. Although the voices disappeared in the fourth year, it could be that they may come back in the event of problems. This is because Daisy's voices make her aware of her problems.

THESE STORIES SHOW …

- first of all that voice hearing can be an unpleasant experience, but you can learn to deal with it;
- that it is an experience that can change over time and that it is related to what happens to you and how you react to this;
- that voices react to your emotions and these emotions are linked to the problems or a trauma you experienced;
- that you need to learn to talk about it, both about the voices and your problems;
- that things will get better when you develop emotionally too, learning to deal with your fear, anger, sadness, etc.;
- that it is important that you receive your parents' support and that you do not become or remain the odd one out at home or at school;
- that you should not give the voices too much power, leaving you feeling much weaker than they are;
- that venting your anger on others as a reaction to the voices does not help in trying to get support. It is better to stop and think about what has made you so angry;
- that psychiatrists who do not accept your voices are no use to you. Medication on its own does not help;
- that you can decide that there is no room for voices in your life any more.

Pete's Story

Pete's mother phoned in response to the advertisement about the congress for children hearing voices that we organised in Amsterdam in 1993. She wanted to attend the congress with Pete. He was not doing well, particularly at school. He was obstinate, did not want to study and did not feel the need to conform to any kind of system whatsoever. On the whole, he was an insecure, scared 15-year-old who did not know what he wanted to do in the future.

Pete started hearing voices when he was 6, after his family had moved house. At that time, Kim, a four-year-old girl who was a classmate of Pete's brother, James, died. For a while, Pete took a rose to Kim's mother every single day. Death made Pete insecure, and he would often come home to his mother crying. When he was six, Pete was treated for a year by a child psychologist because of his fear of death. When we met him he was being treated by a child psychiatrist because of his voices. Pete's mother consented to us contacting this psychiatrist in order to ask him whether he wanted to give a lecture at our congress about Pete's story. This psychiatrist had accepted Pete's voices and was interested in Pete's experiences. After the children's congress in 1993 the voices disappeared.

Pete heard three voices that others could not hear. He heard them in his head and did not think that he, himself, was the voice. He was able to talk to the voices. Pete heard the voice of 'a granddad', another male voice and a female voice. Granddad had been the previous inhabitant of Pete's house and had hanged himself above the stairs. Granddad was wise and positive. He challenged Pete to little games to see whether Pete could win. The female voice was an unfamiliar voice of a woman of around 40 years old. The third voice was unfamiliar too and ageless. Both these voices could be positive or negative. Granddad would comment on the negative voice. For example, when Pete was unsure about whether to get off his bike or cycle on, the negative voice said: 'Cycle on'. Then the voice of granddad said: 'Why don't you stop?' Pete did not listen to his granddad, but cycled on and had an accident.

The voices offered advice, offered solutions to problems, criticised, forbade things, made him angry, sometimes talked through his conversations and interrupted pleasant activities. They often set tasks. Pete was scared of the voices. They upset him and disturbed his daily life. They made Pete powerless. The voices were in control. Pete was passive when he started hearing voices. He did not do anything and mainly remained scared of them.

The voices would typically appear when Pete was scared. The voices would talk to him at school when he had to do an exam. They would say: 'Just give up, you won't pass, just go and do something else'. According to Pete the things the voices said often had something to do with his own desires. 'For example, I did not want to do that exam anyway. If I want to do something else other than what the voices tell me to do, then I do what I want to do myself and not what the voices want me to do.'

This was not easy, since the negative voices could also be threatening. They said that if Pete did not carry out their tasks, an accident would happen – his mother would die. Pete did not give in to the threats of the voices – he noticed that they threatened, but they were not necessarily right.

Pete did not feel safe at school. He was bullied, attacked and he was regularly sworn at too. Pete also had the feeling that he was the odd one out. Pete was very insecure and would often blame himself when something was not going right.

An incident which, according to Pete's mother, has been of influence on their family life and Pete's development was the fact that she found out that she had been sexually abused when she was young. She was 36 when she found out and Pete was 10 at that time. Following this, his mother had undergone psychiatric treatment for a while.

Our next meeting was a couple of years later. By now, Pete was 18. From a lanky teenager he had developed into a great big man. Pete had just graduated from his marine training. He had a steady girlfriend and exuded confidence. However, Pete was hearing voices again.

Pete was hearing the voice of an unfamiliar, ageless man. This had started during the intense marine training course and the extremely tough physical training. Pete was not that scared of the voice. Pete could send him away and talk to him. He would sometimes swear at him, sometimes out loud, sometimes in his head. He could refuse the tasks. He could call up the voice and shut himself off from it. The voice did not disturb his daily life any more.

Pete had the feeling that he was in control of the voice. That had happened after he had to retake a year at school and he had started thinking about his future and suddenly he knew what he wanted: to make money.

Pete had also become more proactive. He could send the voice away, ignore it, listen, listen selectively, distract his thoughts and set limits. He was able to do other things, go and see someone, seek distraction and carry out rituals. Everything helped. He would usually listen critically to the things the voice said and then he would make a decision about it. Sometimes this worked, sometimes it did not. According to Pete, the voice was more of a good guide or was the voice linked to his paranormal gift?

After our conversation Pete very kindly took me to the station on his bike, so that I would be in time to catch my train. Following our conversation, the voice disappeared and did not return again that year. This surprised Pete.

At our next meeting, a year later, Pete told me that during the previous year he had been sent to Bosnia for three months. He had, in fact, expected to start hearing voices again when he was confronted with death there. Right in front of his own eyes one of the mine disposal team stepped on an anti-tank mine. Pete had been talking to him just before he walked to his death. Pete and the others had to collect the remains of this man in a bag. Pete thought that the fact that the voices stayed away had to do with his own decision that he did not want to hear them any more.

The following year Pete had started living with his girlfriend. When he went with me to my car at the end of the interview, I was shown an example of his professional training. Just beyond my car there was a bit of trouble and a policeman was involved. He was trying to arrest someone who was resisting. Pete did not hesitate for a moment and jumped in to help the policeman. He got hold of this stocky man and slammed him against the wall with one blow, so that he could keep both the man's arms spread. The man was standing there powerless. When the policeman tried to handcuff the man, things went wrong again and he tried to escape. Again Pete intervened. He pulled the man to the ground and they were both rolling about. With the help of the policeman, Pete managed to get the man's hands behind his back. After the man had been handcuffed, Pete yanked him up. The man did not flinch, but when he was standing he said: 'Mind my glasses; they are on the ground'. Pete let go of the man, picked up the glasses and put these on the man's nose and joined the rest of the onlookers. When I drove off I saw three police cars with wailing sirens coming towards me.

During our last meeting there were few changes. The only thing that had changed was that Pete had a new girlfriend and he was living at home again, awaiting a new home. His contract with the marines was due to expire at the end of the month and Pete did not want to extend it as it would mean that he would be away from home a lot. He was negotiating a job with KLM. He would join the anti-terror team and would accompany difficult passengers on their flights where he would have to get involved if there was any trouble. It sounded good to him.

Pete did not hear any voices any more. He developed an inner dialogue and used this to put things into perspective. Reflecting on his experiences, Pete said that it had mainly been his fear of the voices that had inhibited him. As a result of his profession, he had learned to deal with fear in a completely different way. 'Fear disappears much quicker than you think' he said. At work, he had to concentrate and could not have the distraction of the voices. Nobody knew about it anyway. He was worried that if someone knew about it, he would perhaps be dismissed.

However, Pete had not forgotten his experiences. A little girl next door heard the voice of her dead granny in her bedroom. It scared her. Pete visited her in her bedroom. He saw the voice, granny, sitting in the corner and he told the granny out loud that she should not scare the little girl. Since that moment, the girl has not been bothered by the voice.

Paula's Story

Paula had been hearing voices for almost a year. She was ten years old now. It started with two voices talking at the same time. The voices had started a couple of days after her brother's friend, Steve (15 years old), had very suddenly passed away. Steve spent a lot of time at Paula's house. He had been there the evening before his death. He had organised a leaving party as he was moving house and was returning the next day to help clear up. Around eleven o'clock they were called to say he wouldn't be coming, because he had been found dead in his bed. The cause of death was not known. When the cause of death is not known, as a rule an autopsy has to take place. That took a couple of days and because of this, they could only bury Steve two weeks later. Even then the cause of death was not known.

Paula had been confronted before with a sudden death. When she was two, her granny had died totally unexpectedly without having been ill. Granny lived opposite and Paula saw her all the time. Granny's passing away was an incomprehensible event and the sudden death of Steve seemed a repeat of this. In the week of Steve's death Paula ran a very high fever. At night she went to the loo and saw a man behind the bathroom door. Following this the voices started, though one disappeared again the next day.

During our first interview, Paula told me that she heard an evil, angry voice; a 'non-human being'. The tone was mixed, though usually angry. The voice was within her head. She heard the voice almost all day. She did not recognise the voice. She also said: 'It's definitely someone else's, as otherwise I would recognise the voice as my voice.'

Paula also heard creaking, thumping and squeaking. She saw scary faces, skeletons with their heads under their arms and dead, headless bodies. If she was woken up by a sound, she saw the faces of these bodies on the wall or the ceiling. At the same time she would also hear a voice. The voice would appear at night as well as during the day.

Paula was very scared of the voice and she would only feel safe in the living room at home. The voice particularly reinforced her negative feelings and made her angrier, more scared and jealous and would appear when she was bored. The voice would tease and scare her then by talking about skeletons.

The voice would also appear when she was doing pleasant things. He would say: 'Can't you do something else?' He also forbade her to play chess with her dad; something she really enjoyed. When she was watching a quiz on TV, the voice would say: 'If you don't answer ten questions correctly, I'll scare you' and that is indeed what he did by showing her scary skeletons at night. The voice made her have arguments with her brother. He made her feel very insecure by telling her she was doing things wrong. It would give Paula a strange feeling. The voice also commented that the tablets Paula took were 'unnecessary' and also on things her father, mother or brother did.

Paula was afraid to go to bed as she was scared of encountering the skeletons. Each night before she went to bed, her father would come up to her room to check for skeletons and when he assured her they were not there, she would go to sleep relieved.

Because of the voice Paula did things for which she would get punished such as talking out loud to the voice during a lesson at school. She would sometimes hurt someone because the voice had told her to. When she was thinking about something the voice would be thinking at the same time and that confused her. At school it could sometimes be such a pain, as he would mix up all the figures during maths. When he was confusing her, the teacher thought that she was not paying attention. At a certain point the teacher punished her by putting her right at the back of the class. Paula was slightly deaf and could not follow the lesson at all any more. It provided her with lots of time for the voice and that was, of course, a big problem.

The voice preferred to make everything scary. He exploited the burglary at the house of her granddad, who lived on the other side of the street. He scared Paula by explaining exactly how the burglars had got in. Because of this, Paula became very vigilant and every stranger entering her street was regarded as a potential burglar.

Because of the image and the voice Paula did not dare go into her own room any more. Someone would always have to come with her to check her room for scary things. Paula received a lot of support at home. On the advice of her GP, Paula was treated by a child psychiatrist. He prescribed medication for her fear and explained that the voices might be related to Steve's death. Paula did not have any friends her own age. She was bullied a lot at school.

By the time of our next encounter all kinds of things had happened and another story in which death played a role emerged. It turned out that Paula's father, not long after Steve's death, had lost his job. Her mother found the dismissal unfair and got so upset about it that she developed severe heart problems and there was concern for her life. Paula could not deal with this. As her mother would describe later: 'I could not deal with her voices, nor could she with my heart problems'.

During the previous year, Paula's granddad suddenly passed away. He had lived opposite and she had had a close relationship with him. She saw him on an almost daily basis. Paula's mother told me that Paula had dealt with his passing away well. She was given extra attention at that time. Although the voices commented, they were not extra-active. It was unusual that, since his passing away, Paula had hardly, if at all, talked about her granddad. She said: 'I will never forget memories of death, but I will forget all the other things. The voices help me remember death.'

At school the bullying had gotten out of hand. Paula's mother had complained several times to the headteacher and when that did not work she filed a complaint with the school inspectors.

By now, Paula had started to hear one more voice than in the previous year. She heard two male voices of ghosts who were ageless. They did not resemble anybody, but Paula wondered whether one of the ghosts had come from one of the people who had died in her home. The voices talked about Paula and other ghosts.

During the previous year a lot had happened, but the situation with the voices had not improved. The voices appeared more frequently and with more emotions such as anger and fear, but also sadness and jealousy. Paula was still very scared of the voices and they made her even more scared because of their threats. When she felt insecure, the voices would say: 'You simply cannot do it'. When she was in love: 'You should not pick him'. The voices forced her to make decisions. If, in the bathroom, she could choose between a pink and a blue shampoo bottle, the voices forced her to take blue whereas she prefers pink. Paula reacted very passively to the voices. She mainly let her fear dominate and did nothing to set any limits.

The voices took more power and forbade Paula to finish her sentences, which confused her an awful lot. When the voices irritated Paula, she would start picking fights, both at home and at school. Since she answered the voices out loud at school, everybody in her class knew she was hearing a voice and she got bullied even more. But Paula had made a friend by now, a girl from India who was three years her junior and who lived in her street. This girl was very wise. She taught Paula that she should not react to the voice. She illustrated this by saying that she did not react when Paula was trying to pick a fight. Paula put her advice into practice. It worked.

In the following year, the tension surrounding Paula's father unemployment had disappeared. He had found a job. Her mother's symptoms improved. The problems at school had been resolved as it turned out that the three girls who had been bullying Paula had been taken out of school at the beginning of the new school year.

Paula kept on hearing one voice: a male voice of unknown age who said nasty things in a deep voice. To Paula this was not a ghost like the previous year. The voice did not sound like anybody. The voice appeared less often and with fewer emotions, but still with fear, doubt and anger when she felt bad and when she was in love. He did not appear with jealousy any more. He would sometimes set her tasks. Paula was now the only thing the voice talked about.

However, the relationship with the voice had changed. Paula felt more in control. The voice was slightly less negative. He occasionally listened to her, but made her less scared and sometimes gave advice. When she did not do the tasks he had set her, she did not react. At one point she had even called up the voice and that was quite fun, but at the same time scary, so much so that she preferred not to repeat it.

Paula had become proactive. When she heard the voice, she would look for distraction, doing something like cycling, go-karting or visiting a friend. She was able to do this as she felt safer outside on the street.

At our last encounter, Paula told me that she did not hear any voices any more. Things were going really well at school. She had several girlfriends now and she was in love.

John's Story

John's mother read about our study in the paper and decided to take part. John was nine at the time and heard voices. When I visited John for our first interview, his father was at home too. He had fractured both heels and observed the conversation with his son, very quietly and with a lot of interest, from the sofa.

John was the problem child in the family. The parents had looked for help three times. The problems had started when he was a toddler aged two. He was hyperactive. They looked for help from a Catholic healthcare organisation. When John was six, problems at school started and school support advisors were called in. The following year, John started hearing voices and his GP referred him to a child psychiatrist. The term schizophrenia was mentioned. The psychiatrist forbade John and his parents to talk about the voices. He prescribed medication. Initially Dipiperon, but because of the Dipiperon, John would eat all the time. He was prescribed Ritalin next. John has been taking this for two years now.

When I asked my interview question about the nature of his treatment, it felt like I was opening a can of worms. Both parents were angry and very dissatisfied. They were particularly angry at the way the doctor reacted when they asked his advice about the medication. They would phone him when John's behaviour changed either when things were getting worse or when things were getting better. Mother: 'It then feels like they are experimenting with our John. On the phone the doctor just said: "Why don't you add another drop or take a drop less?" He didn't ask whether the drugs were really working. No appointment was made to come and see him. John is just being treated over the telephone.' During our conversation John's parents didn't really discuss his problems at school and that had been the real reason why they had started looking for more information and decided to participate in the research.

John heard the voices of two strangers; he did not know how old they were. One voice was a negative male voice and the other a positive female voice. John: 'They are other people, as there is nobody in my room.' When he was lying in bed, John would see large hyenas and lions with long manes and large, long claws. At the same time he would hear voices, John would also hear sounds like the sound of a garden gate opening, without there being one nearby. He could not talk to the voices.

John remembered how it all started very well. When he was drawing a car, a male voice said: 'You should not draw a car like that'. Two days later he heard a female voice too. According to John, there was no single event that could have been the trigger for his voice hearing, but he was having serious problems at school.

The voices would appear at school and when he was on his own in his room. They would sometimes wake him up. He would get scared and make a racket. That caused problems since it would wake up John's parents. They would come into his room and talk to him. He had to stay in his own room. They would let him keep the door ajar and in the corridor they would switch on a nightlight.

The voices would appear when John was angry and when he was scared. They would appear when he was sad, '... when I've lost something ...'; when he was tired and did not know what to do. The voices reinforced John's negative feelings.

It was particularly at school that the voices would follow a certain pattern. The female voice would give him advice in a friendly way, followed by the male voice commenting on this. The man and the woman would then start an argument and that is how they confused John. The voices would appear when he was doing maths, history, geography, art and road safety lessons.

The voices made John easily irritated and then he would start fights. John did not have any real friends. There were regular problems because of John's aggression. He would often pick fights in a self-defeating way; picking fights with boys who he knew beforehand that he could not beat, since they were stronger. John's father told me that this behaviour had been the reason why they had made John give up the football club. He would start picking fights with his team-mates in the dressing room.

According to John's mother, John cannot cope with change, which is why the family strictly adheres to a regular schedule. 'If, in the evening, he knows that things will be different the next day, then things begin to go wrong.' The voices have led to the family living according to a regular routine.

John liked talking about his experiences. Afterwards he wanted to show me his school which was around the corner.

Not long after our meeting, John's parents found a different therapist. John is being treated by the same GP as David now. This doctor started by gradually weaning him off the Ritalin that had been prescribed by his psychiatrist. Following that, he drew up an inventory list of John's symptoms and their link to his daily life. He prescribed John homeopathic drugs. John started sleeping much better and became far less aggressive. After two months the voices disappeared, and at the same time John's school performance deteriorated. He was tested and it turned out he had an IQ of 85. John was immediately placed on the waiting list for a school that suited his academic abilities much better. John's mother told me that his teachers reported to her that John would often overestimate himself and certain situations. John did not have a sense of reality and as an example, the teacher said that when they had to solve a maths question about the speed of a cyclist, John calculated that the cyclist was travelling at a speed of 150 miles per hour.

'Is that possible?' the teacher asked.

'Why not?' John answered.

When we met next, the voices had disappeared. John had changed schools and, in order to get there, he had to go by bus to another village. That went well.

When John's problems were taken into consideration, his mother noticed that he got into fewer fights. Therefore he slept better and the tension at home reduced too. John's mother would lovingly stroke him on his head and say: 'He may not be hearing any voices anymore, but I don't know how he is going to earn his money with an IQ of 85.'

'Baker', John promptly replied.

'That's possible as we don't have a baker in the family yet', his mother replied. 'You can't become a tiler, as your father is a tiler already.' When I left, the whole family waved me off, father, mother with John on one side and his sister on the other. I had to turn my car around, so

I had a good view. His little sister bent over and stuck her tongue out at John. When he did not react, she did it again and this time John got really angry. The parents, who had only seen John's reaction, but not the trigger, immediately punished John. Shame they could not have seen it from my position.

During our last interview John told me that occasionally he hears a voice again. His mother, who did not know this, was shocked. John is not scared of the voice. The voice does not really say proper words, but just flashes past. John still finds it difficult to talk about his emotions. His parents now give him more attention when emotional things happen, such as when his six-year-old niece died last year and the entire family was crying at the funeral, but John had not cried. He said that he could not cry and his mother had talked to him about that in more depth.

About daily emotions: at night, John is sometimes scared, but he keeps his bedroom door ajar then. This works. He regularly feels guilty. Now he is in love. During the course of the study John made more friends. He has also found a hobby that suits him. He is completely into his drums and together with a couple of friends he has formed a band.

His mother told us that the voices doctor had discovered that chocolate made John aggressive. He cannot have that any more. She is very happy that she took part in the study and, as a result, she feels supported to deal with her son's voices in a different way. She watched a programme on TV during the week in which the voices are labelled as a disease and schizophrenic. She was livid about this. She said: 'These people are dangerous, they make children ill – look what they almost did to our John. We were not allowed to talk about the voices and all he got was drugs.'

David's Story

David's foster mother phoned to make an appointment. She was concerned about David who heard voices. She had been to two different healthcare organisations, but neither of them was able to answer her questions properly. The word schizophrenia was mentioned and she was shocked about this. She did not want to go in that direction. By taking part in the study, she wanted to obtain more information about voice hearing. She knew that we would not medicate.

When I entered the cosy living room, David, a bit like a toddler, was playing with toddler's wooden toys. He had hidden himself behind the sofa. The conversation was difficult. It was not easy for David to talk about his experiences either. During our conversation he went to sit on his foster mother's lap. She reacted patiently and sweetly and allowed him to be the little child that just wanted to be cuddled.

David is 13 years old. He started hearing voices six years ago. He was seven at the time. The problems started when his parents divorced. David was three at the time and, together with his younger brother, went to live with his mother. The mother was not settled. David moved house at least ten times. His mother remarried when David was five years old.

David was regularly abused by his mother and stepfather. It started with swearing and hitting and it ended with locking him up for hours in the garden shed. After the first time he had been locked up he started hearing voices.

Two years ago he was taken away from his mother. Initially he and his younger brother were going to live with his father, but he could not take on caring for the boys as he had a full-time job. His father sought help and that is how David and his brother came to live with foster parents during the week and at weekends with their dad. David started regarding his foster parents as 'father' and 'mother' and called the others his 'biological mother and father'. David had no friends.

David heard ten voices of people he knew well – of his biological mother, her current husband, of his biological father and a whole series of relatives – most relatives were from his biological mother's side. All voices were negative. He heard them every day. He could not talk to them. David heard knocking sounds and, in the evening, he would sometimes see shadows.

David heard the voices during the day and at night. Emotions were triggers. The voices were happy when David was sad or scared. They reinforced certain emotions. They appeared when he felt insecure. When he felt guilty, they tried to reinforce that feeling, when he felt unhappy they would say 'Great!' When he felt alone they would say 'We are your friends'. They reinforced his feelings of embarrassment. They would appear when he was tired. So the voices were always nasty and they would harass him.

The voices would also exploit his insecurity during the period in which he learned to trust his new mother. They would forbid him to make friends with her: 'Don't talk to her!' or they would say 'Why don't you leave that cow?' They would swear at him.

The voices had an enormous impact and dominated David's daily life. David was scared and felt as if he had been made powerless. The voices set tasks and David had to obey. If he did so, the voices were nice. The tasks could go really far, such as chasing his brother with a knife. The voices confused him and caused an inability to concentrate well, which meant he could not pay attention at school do any homework. The voices were never helpful; they were mainly negative. Therefore, David just found them nasty.

His foster mother asked me for the name of a therapist who could treat David, but who would not just give him a psychiatric diagnosis. I advised a homeopathic doctor who treated children who heard voices. The homeopathic doctor prescribed magnesium silicate for David and it helped him keep his aggression more under control. He took these every other day. David's foster mother said that she noticed every time he needed them again.

When we met for the second time, David had changed a lot. He said: 'I feel confident about life again' and that was new. He had developed his muscles and had lost his 'puppy fat'. Also, I did not have to make an effort to establish contact with him. He was no longer the needy child of the previous year. David had discovered that he was a talented cyclist. His foster parents were very enthusiastic and bought him a beautiful bike. He started winning cycling races. His foster mother offered 100 per cent support to David. Day and night she was available on her mobile. However, this did not mean that she accepted everything in terms of behaviour. There were clear limits.

David still heard the same voices. Although the voices themselves had not changed and, like the previous year, had a great influence on his life, David found that the voices were less negative and had less impact. Whereas twelve months earlier, David had been scared of the voices, now he reacted by getting angry at them. He said: 'I have more courage now and I can do more. I feel much better inside.' David was able to talk to the voices and sometimes they reacted. If he said 'Go away!' they would answer: 'You must be joking'. However, if he then replied: 'I'm going to pray' they would say, 'OK!' and disappear.

Moreover, David did not always have to do the things the voices told him to do any more. Generally speaking, David found that he was more in control. He was the boss – he would say – since the voices were in his head.

During our conversation, it was noticeable that he had become more objective. He pushed aside his feelings a bit more. David still did not have any friends. He was not ready to deal with his past. He preferred to bury everything that reminded him of the past.

The following year both David's foster mother and his younger brother Nicolas became very ill. There was a lot of tension and serious differences of opinion between David's foster parents and David's biological father about David and Nicolas's upbringing. Legally nothing had been laid down about the rights and duties of both parties. The adults had their problems, but for the boys this conflict was a problem too. They would run away to their father, but that did not go well. The boys were allowed to return to their foster parents if they made a clear choice. Both boys decided in favour of the foster parents. Their foster mother could not cope with all the stress and she started to suffer from heart rhythm problems and had to have heart surgery.

In that year Nicolas suddenly began to suffer from paralysis in his legs and he was admitted to hospital. His foster mother paid a lot of attention to Nicolas and David became jealous. The voices reacted to the problems and became more dominant. David talked to them and told them 'Go away!' and then the voice would say, 'We are simply not going'. Very rarely was he able to refuse tasks. David was not able to shut himself off from the voices, but was not overwhelmed by fear either any more. According to David, both he and the voices were boss.

David may have wanted to be in control of the voices, but the influence of the voices in his daily life had increased. They told him to play truant and to be violent at school. David was punished more and more. He reacted to this by pushing away all his emotions. David could not care less about anyone any more; he did not care about the punishments either. At school and at home he was hardly manageable and his foster mother told me that she was not sure how long she could go on like this. At the time of our meeting, there was talk of David having to leave home and school.

After our conversation, David's foster mother consulted their GP. He contacted us and asked for the study data. He did not know that David had been abused and that voice hearing could be a reaction to that. He subsequently referred David to a psychiatric consultation because of the voices. The voices were regarded as functional and not psychotic. His foster mother was advised to send him to a boarding school as he had difficulty with closeness.

When we had our last interview, several things had changed. On the advice of a therapist, David was sent to a boarding school in Belgium. He did not like the first one. After a few months he moved to a boarding school which specialised in training cyclists. It's a stricter school and David liked it. He went home at weekends. David's brother Nicolas ran away to this father again. There was no contact any more. According to David, Nicolas had started taking drugs.

The voices had reacted favourably to these events. David still heard the same voices, but less often. The voices would still appear with his emotions, but David had learned to talk about them in a better way now. He had learned to control his anger better, which had caused problems before. According to David this was due to the tough physical training he had to endure because of the cycling.

The relationship with the voices had become more balanced. If David told the voices 'Piss off!' they would indeed disappear. So they listened to him. They would only agree with him if he did things that were clearly not acceptable. He did not give the voices the chance to set more tasks for him. However, he sometimes believed what the voices said and then he would simply agree with them.

Despite all his problems, David was doing really well. He looked like a real hunk with his bleached hair. He told me that he had made a number of decisions. He had decided to be nicer to his foster mother, to care for her, as things were difficult enough for her. David was able to feel his emotions again – something he had not been able to do the previous year. David had gained wisdom about life and I heard him advise his foster mother how she should behave towards her family. He had also decided to make the most of things at school. He was in love, but was also walking around with the picture of another girl in his pocket. He was still a passionate cyclist.

Two years later I phoned David's foster mother again. She told me he was doing really well. His voices had disappeared and he was taking part in cycle races.

Emily's Story

Emily's mother phoned me after she had read about our study in the newspaper. She really wanted Emily to take part. Emily was 15 years old and lived with her parents. She had a steady boyfriend. Things were not going too well for her. Emily heard voices, suffered from obsessive compulsive behaviour and was being treated for that. The therapist was talking about an admission to hospital, something her mother wanted to avoid. Emily had left school, as the voices had too much influence on her thinking.

Emily used to be the perfect child. There were never any problems and she would always obey her parents. Emily started hearing voices when she was seven, after a classmate had told her that God would punish you if you did not listen to him. Emily heard a male voice who threatened to punish her if she did not listen. So, from the very beginning, Emily obeyed this voice unconditionally. In this way Emily avoided all conflicts.

Around the age of 10, the male voice changed into a girl's voice. At that time Emily witnessed an argument between her mother and her sister, Pia, which got out of hand. Pia and her mother had an argument in the kitchen during which Pia's mother forbade Pia, who was 14, to have any contact with her older boyfriend. She thought Pia too young for that. Pia, completely in love, did not agree and got hold of a kitchen knife with which she threatened her own mother. Emily and her mother never talked about this event again. Her mother was embarrassed about it too.

Around the age of 12, Emily started to suffer from obsessive compulsive behaviour and eating disorders. (Obsessive compulsive behaviour usually develops from a need to control one's life.)

When she was 14 Emily was sexually abused. She started hearing another voice, a girl of her own age, a positive voice that supported her.

During our first meeting, Emily described her experience: 'The voices sit in a large, white room and I am sitting there too, but I cannot see the voices.' Other people could not hear the voices. She thought that the voices were other people, but she was worried that the voices could be from inside her as well. We talked more in-depth about her experience and Emily admitted that the voices were of others who were in her head. She was able to talk to the voices.

Emily heard the voices of two girls of her age, 14 or 15. One voice was negative, the other positive. The negative voice set Emily tasks all day, usually repeating what she had already done, like, for instance, the hoovering. The positive voice supported and comforted her by saying: 'Don't listen to it!' The negative voice blackmailed her and told Emily that if she did not listen her mother would die. Both voices wanted Emily to like them: '... as otherwise we will start to hate you' they said.

The negative voice would appear when Emily was scared, sad, jealous, guilty or when she felt ashamed and also when she was bored. The voice would then aggravate her emotions in a negative way. The voices would appear in negative situations when Emily felt insecure. It is interesting to see that the voices mainly appeared in times of stress and they would make Emily's insecurity worse. Over time, they stopped her doing anything.

The voices were present most of the day. They would scare Emily. But when the voices disappeared, she would immediately be scared in anticipation of the moment they would come back again. As a result, Emily herself filled her entire day with fear.

Emily would regularly be so scared of the voices during the day that she would suffer from physical reactions such as headaches or feeling tight-chested. Most of the day she would feel depressed. She would then go to bed and sleep a lot which irritated most of the other family members. She had lost all interest in life and was not eating well. Emily didn't question, she completely gave in to them. She felt powerless.

In the year between our first and second meeting, all kinds of things happened. An admission to a psychiatric hospital could not be avoided, but the treatment did not work. Two months in hospital caused Emily to be very angry and to decide that she never wanted to be admitted again.

Emily continued with her life and was looking forward. She decided that she would not return to her secondary school but, instead, follow a vocational course. She decided to train as a hairdresser. At this school she did not have any homework and she spent less hours at school. She suffered less from the voices.

However, the change did not seem to work. At our next meeting, Emily had left her hairdresser's training. It just did not work, too much stress. Emily looked for help and started following a course which was aimed at learning to deal with depression. She recognised her problems and did not think she was suffering from the worst problems and was satisfied with the course. Her mother followed the parent part of this course and was very enthusiastic about it. She understood Emily better.

Following that, Emily went to work in a supermarket. At our last meeting, it turned out that she was not working there at all any more. After her supermarket job, she had worked as a sales assistant in a shoe shop for a while, but here too, the voices interfered too much with her work, so she gave up. She was tested and was advised to follow an administrative training course. Given her voices, this was not very realistic advice for Emily.

Compared with the first meeting, we saw positive changes in Emily. She had learned how to deal with her emotions in a better way. She suffered less from obsessive compulsive behaviour. She did not sleep as much as before. At home there were fewer arguments. Emily's entire family had accepted her voices, but would hardly ever talk about them.

Emily said, 'Nobody is occupied 24 hours a day with them, like in the beginning. At that time, all we talked about was me. Now it is more normal. I'm not an exception any more.'

The drawback was that Emily had obeyed the voices too much and had handed over too much control to them. She had tried too hard to avoid anything which made her feel insecure and had limited her activities too much. She just sat at home most of the time. She was still hearing voices, but quite liked these. It meant she was not so alone then. The voices had, in fact, achieved everything that she had wanted to achieve when they appeared for the first time – avoiding stress and conflict in daily life. They limited Emily's insecurity since hardly any surprises ever happened, now that she stayed at home all day without a skill. Since the frequency of the voices had lessened, Emily was able to move around the house more freely. In addition, she does not suffer from daily depression anymore.

However, there was a downside to this seemingly good compromise. Emily had manoeuvred herself into a very vulnerable position. She did not have a job any more. She had lost her girlfriends. She was not careful with the contacts she still had. She could be very unreasonable to her parents and boyfriend when she was angry and that happened regularly. Emily was looking forward to moving in with her boyfriend. She did not have any other future expectations apart from living together. Her mother was concerned and wondered how long her boyfriend would cope and, if there was no boyfriend anymore, what would happen then?

Ben's Story

Ben's mother heard about our study on the radio and decided to take part. Ben was 11 and heard voices. She herself did not dare to talk to Ben about his experiences. His behaviour caused a lot of problems, both at home and at school. His parents had reached the point where they did not know how to deal with him any more. However, going to a psychiatrist was just that step too far. They were trying to control Ben by setting rules, but that did not work and it made Ben even more of a problem.

During our first meeting Ben did not want to have anything to do with me. He sat on the other side of the sofa on the armrest to make it clear to me that he could walk out at any time he liked. His father had taken an afternoon off especially for this meeting. Both parents were interested to follow what Ben and I were doing. I put my box of tricks on the table: my computer with games. Ben's objections melted away like the snow in the sun and he came and sat next to me full of interest. After he had played a game, he was prepared to talk about his voices.

Ben had started hearing voices when he was six. Initially, it started with scary images and, following that, came the voices. According to Ben, there was no particular reason for it at all. It just started one day. The only thing Ben remembered about that time was that he was madly in love with a girl, but she was not interested. In that same period, his granddad has passed away.

Ben heard between four and ten male, female and children's voices in his head, which he thought were not him. Sometimes he doubted whether or not these were his own thoughts.

Ben saw images regularly. For example, when he went to the video shop with his friend, he would see pictures of scary faces. In the evening the faces returned as people and he saw them walking around in his room. With street fights the background could blur and he would sometimes see someone who stood in between the two people who were fighting. Ben heard thumping and sometimes felt touches. Ben had premonitions which made him feel powerless. For example, he would know beforehand that he would get into an argument and to him that meant having a problem. 'When I get into a fight, I never dare to hit back.'

The male and female voices changed with Ben's moods. When Ben was nice, the voices were nice too; when he was angry, the voices were angry too. He only liked the children's voices as they invited him to come and play with them. The voices appeared at home, at school and in the street. The main trigger was arguments or fights. According to Ben, school fights moved to his head. 'If I have an argument with someone, I think, "I am the one in the middle here".' At night he would see the school in his head and hear the voices of monsters. The voice would appear when Ben was angry or scared and when he felt guilty.

Ben was scared of the voices. The voices decided what Ben was allowed to say and what not to say. Most of the time he was not allowed to talk about the voices. They could also tell him to talk, but they would first tell what he had to say. For example; 'You are allowed to say something. Why don't you tell your friend that he is a queer?' This is what Ben did and, of course, they would have an argument.

However, Ben was able to talk to the voices. He would say: 'Piss off! I hate you!' or: 'I will kill you!' and then the voices would answer: 'Try it, you won't succeed'.

Unfortunately, the introduction part of our meeting had taken up so much of our time that we were not finished with the research interview when it was supper time. A new meeting had to be scheduled. When Ben saw me off at the door, I could hear two girls on the other side of the road swearing at Ben. At first they had not noticed that I was standing behind Ben. As soon as they realised that, they walked on. Ben told me that these girls were his sister and her friend. His sister never caused any problems at home. Ben's parents were much nicer to her, she was never punished. What his parents did not see was that the sister was secretly bullying Ben. In all kinds of ways, she showed him that she could not stand him. Ben himself did not have any real friends.

When I returned three weeks later to finish the interview, it seemed as if I had come to a totally different family. A bomb had exploded. In the living room, a stocky man with a lot of muscles, not the father, was walking around. The mother did not explain an awful lot, but in between the lines I understood what was happening here. This man turned out to be a friend of the family who was helping them to get Ben on the straight and narrow again. From Ben I understood that Ben had been testing their patience too much. He had set fire to things and tried to jump from a block of flats. Enough was enough.

I had agreed to meet Ben at 4pm, but he was not home. He had been home briefly, but when his mother had discovered that he had not written down his homework, she sent him back to school to get it. That was 45 minutes ago and the school was around the corner. After a short conversation, the family friend went to look for Ben. He found him in the schoolyard, where he was playing with his friends. When he went back to school, it was closed. Ben still did not know what kind of homework he had to do and he had forgotten his date with me.

His mother was furious and punished him by sending him to his room. I had to follow him for our conversation. Ben was not impressed. Ben's room was full of Ninja posters. Ben enthusiastically showed me all kinds of fighting positions whilst explaining this combat sport. During our conversation I noticed how straight Ben was.

'Do you ever lie?' was one of the questions in the questionnaires.

'Yes,' admitted Ben wholeheartedly, 'regularly.'

'Do you ever steal?'

'Yes,' said Ben, without hesitation.

Very few children in the study were able to be this honest. Such honestly commonly leads to problems with others.

His mother did not turn out to be that bad. After fifteen minutes she brought up some soft drinks, but she remained angry with Ben. When we returned downstairs, she told him to go to school at 8am the following day in order to do his homework there. Ben shrugged his shoulders in a resigned way and disappeared to his room.

Therefore I was able to ask his mother another couple of questions. Because of all Ben's stories about fighting I asked her whether she would allow him to start doing some sports. It turned out that Ben had done judo in the past, but could not cope with the theoretical part of it.

Both parents were convinced that theoretical stuff was a problem for Ben. He was someone who learned by doing things. They hoped he would go to agricultural college the following year, where he could work with his hands.

At the next meeting, Ben himself opened the front door. He had been waiting for me. Compared to the previous year, there was a totally different atmosphere in the house. Ben's mother walked around radiantly and she told me that she had a little job now. Since she was away from home more often, Ben and his sister were on their own more and everyone involved liked that very much. We talked about the past year. How had Ben been getting on? His mother gave very relaxed answers and would sometimes stroke Ben's head with a smile on her face. I saw warmth and intimacy which had not been there the year before. In the living room Ben's sister was watching TV with headphones on. Only the dog had remained aggressive. It growled and went for me twice when Ben's mother went to the kitchen to get coffee for me. I jumped behind the kitchen door just in time to save myself. Ben, himself, chose to have our conversation in his bedroom again. He had changed his room and I was given a tour. There were still a lot of posters and pictures, but this time for girl bands. Girls occupied him day and night.

A lot had changed with his experiences too. Ben heard far fewer voices and they appeared less often. A male voice remained which usually appeared at night. Ben was also less scared of the voices. At school the situation had changed as well. Ben had become popular. Whereas last year he would have been the last one to be chosen for a team game, he was now first. He was not bullied any more either.

A year later, the relationship between Ben and his parents appeared to have become more mature, far more equal now. To give you an example: during the conversation I asked the children whether their parents ever had any arguments and how they dealt with that. When I asked Ben that question both the mother and Ben started laughing. Ben answered the question first: 'If they begin to fight I shout downstairs "Can't you keep your voice down a bit?"' Ben's mother started to roar with laughter. Initially Ben laughed with her, but after a while he said in very strict tone: 'That's enough now'. His mother tried, but that's difficult when you're in stitches.

Ben's behaviour changed, but so had his mother's opinions about his experiences: 'I thought he had more of a gift, like my mother. She was able to predict things that would then happen, but that is not the case with Ben. He has some premonitions, but they don't usually come true. Ben also started doing all these dangerous things.' Since his behaviour was not causing problems anymore, as far as she was concerned an explanation about his exceptional experiences was not relevant any more. 'I am able to help him a lot better now, since I understand his anger problem a lot better now', she said. Ben's parents also took his abilities into account with the choice of school for him. Ben was about to go to secondary school. On the basis of his grades he could have chose a medium-level school. His parents preferred him to take things easy and chose a lower-level school. That would lead to less tension. Furthermore, the lower level school fitted better with the family from a social point of view. 'He can always switch to a higher level', his father said.

The voices disappeared at secondary school when Ben learned to deal with his anger.

During our last meeting, things were going well for Ben. He was getting good grades at school. Talking about the past, Ben was of the opinion that his problems had mainly been at school. At primary school, Ben had fallen out with almost the entire class, whereas he had actually tried to avoid anger. Ben had got himself stuck because of his own reasoning. 'When I get angry, I am so strong, that I can completely beat up the other person. I don't want that.' This reasoning worked liked a boomerang; Ben did not get angry himself, but he would make others angry. During the interviews it emerged that Ben's opinion about his anger had not changed, but he had learned to deal with it in a different way. He had learned that at school with the help of a teacher. After this teacher had witnessed a fight between Ben and a classmate, he called Ben over and asked him for an explanation. Following that, the teacher also invited the other boy to come and have a chat with him. In his presence, Ben and the boy had to explain the reason for their anger with each other. The teacher showed where and how they could come to a compromise. They then had to shake hands and keep their promise. Every time Ben got angry and felt powerless, he asked the teacher to act as a referee during the conversation. That worked.

Ben was able to distance himself from his anger more. He came up with another reason this time, 'Getting angry once can happen and that is allowed,' Ben said, 'but if I get angry about the same thing more often, then it is not my fault, but something else must be the matter. There must be a problem.'

Ben was still scared that he would lose his temper and beat someone up. However, he had thought this out too. He knew by now that he was stronger, since he had done a self-defence course and did some weightlifting. Since he knew what was what, he preferred to turn his back when a fight was brewing and he would walk away. He found that he did not need to prove himself.

Ben did not hear any voices any more, but held an inner dialogue. In case of trouble, he would tell himself: 'Just sit down and don't say anything and then you won't get into trouble.'

During the course of the study, Ben became far happier with life. The young boy who drove his parents to desperation became a knight in shining armour during the course of the study. At our last conversation, we went to his room and Ben took my cup of coffee up the stairs and held the door open for me. When we said our goodbyes, he handed me a bottle of wine wrapped in foil, 'As a thank you', he said.

Laura's Story

Laura was 18 years old. She had heard about our study and decided to take part. When she entered the room I saw an attractive girl with a beautiful, even face and a good figure. She was a little shy, but she put her shyness aside as soon as we began talking about her experiences. That absorbed her, that was what she wanted to talk about.

Things were not going well with Laura. She was on a waiting list for admission, since she could get extremely angry and she would self-harm on a regular basis. Her mother had had enough; she did not want her to stay at home any more.

Laura had been in day-care twice for six months; she did not know why, but not because of the voices. She felt very badly treated: 'I fell out of the frying pan into the fire. The voices were a problem. When I told them that I heard voices, they wanted to know what the voices were telling me. The voices did not allow me to do that. When I did so, they punished me. I told a counsellor about that. Consequently I was given drugs and the counsellors never mentioned the voice again. I didn't get any help, but instead I had one more problem.'

Before I started the interview, I asked Laura to fill in a Dissociative Experiences Scale (DES). The DES is a measuring tool which establishes the measure of dissociation. Dissociation is something that we all do to a certain extent. If we experience something that we do not like, we hide it in our memory in a place where it does not bother us. When you experience very nasty things, as a reaction you may dissociate a great deal. You might, for instance, wake up on a beach and not know how you got there. When you do that, and you do that often, it can cause problems in your daily life. And there is something else too. People with a high dissociative score (above 30) have probably experienced a severe trauma. In that case the voices can be a reaction to the trauma meaning that you have not come to terms with that trauma yet. Laura scored 60.

When Laura was six years old, she started hearing voices (in the same period her grandma passed away). It started at school with a pleasant voice. She was not scared of it, as she thought that hearing voices was normal; that everybody heard voices. Therefore she did not mind that the voice started appearing more and more.

When she was eight, a second voice joined. Just like that, without any particular reason. This voice was pleasant too. Laura spent a lot of time on her own, had few friends and the voices were pleasant company. When she was 12, Laura asked a boy in the schoolyard whether he was hearing voices too. Laura: 'The boy looked at me in such a strange way. He asked whether I was crazy. I was so shocked. I immediately felt like the school idiot. Following that, I started to hear a third voice, a very hostile, nasty voice.' Laura realised that she had an extra world. An 'upper world' as she called it. According to Laura, she had not experienced anything special; there seemed to be no experience of a trauma.

Laura heard one and sometimes two voices now. The voice she heard every day and usually all day long was of a ghost. She called it a ghost as she could not see any clothes. It was a kind of black shadow. She did not recognise the voice.

According to Laura, the voices would always appear by surprise. When she thought about it, it turned out that there were things that could trigger the voices such as the presence of other people. 'I do want to hear the voices. That's why I prefer to be alone. Sometimes I cannot even tolerate my boyfriend near me.' Almost any emotion would trigger the voices: emotions such as fear, anger, sadness and jealousy. The voices could reinforce or slightly weaken the emotions. Laura differentiated between her own emotions and the emotions which trigger the voices.

Fear is an emotion of the voices. Fear usually has to do with my upper world. The voices can make me even more scared or, on the contrary, stimulate me to withdraw. All other emotions are mine. The voices can sometimes interfere in a positive way. For example, when I am angry, they will say that I will have to make it up. When I am sad, they make me even more sad or they comfort me. When I am tired more voices appear.

Then again, the voices are usually nice. They talk about my world. My world is black and white and full of criminals. For example, they say: 'you are the odd one out'. I don't find this negative, as it is a fact. It's only when they talk about my father, mother or sister, I don't listen to them. The voices help and protect me. For example, when I really don't know what to do with my upper world, the voice will tell me how I can get out. That brings peace. Sometimes I think of problems and, next, the voice offers solutions. When, for example, I wonder what things will be like on Earth or Mars if all oxygen had gone, the voice will explain what things will be like. The voice also helps me make decisions, as I cannot choose. When I have to choose, I get totally confused. I cannot even decide between a white or brown sandwich or what I want on it.

Laura may have had a problem with making decisions; the voices did not. They were dictating Laura's choices more and more. 'They want me to wear black clothes and I don't even like black.'

Influence of the voices
The voice of the ghost would sometimes also set tasks which got Laura into trouble. For example, she had to harm herself.

The voice sometimes tells me to steal. He tells me that I need a lot of money for my own world. When I stole money, I got punished. I don't do that any more. In the past he told me to bite people or squeeze the dog. I don't do that any more, as I cannot hurt animals. Furthermore, the voice can confuse me, he tells me what I should and should not think, tells me what I should and should not do, swears at me sometimes, comments on things and he can even make me want to run away. The voice can punish by nagging in my head.

Laura talked to the voice very often; she had discussions with the voice. She talked to it in her thoughts as she found it strange to talk out loud. The voice would listen to her, but only with trivial things would it take her into consideration. For example, when she wanted to phone her boyfriend it would first say 'No!' but later they would give in. When she was alone, Laura would call up the voice. The voices could take 'complete control' of her.

'Who is in control?' I asked.

'I hope it is me, but I think the voice, because he is very strong. He says better things than I do too. He has more life experience.'

The ghost did not allow Laura to repeat all the things he said literally. He threatened to punish her if she did not listen to him. Two years ago he had threatened to cause her father to have an accident if she did not listen. She did not listen and the voice carried out his threat too. It was not a serious accident, just a collision with some damage to the car, but Laura was upset by it.

The voices were worse than the images. She could sometimes really laugh about them. She had more or less become familiar with them and could deal with them, for instance, by taking a break like going to the loo.

I don't want to get rid of the voices. The only thing I really want is to be able to concentrate better and I want get rid of those black spots. In fact, I usually like it when the voices appear, since they talk to me so that I am not alone. Although I am sometimes scared of them, cannot do what I want and they confuse me, I find the voices predominantly positive. I find not being able to do something not as unpleasant as being alone.

Laura indeed was on her own a great deal. She did not go to school and did not have girlfriends. She had one male friend, who was psychiatric patient too. She could talk about her experiences to him.

At our second interview, it turned out that a lot had changed. Laura had been admitted to a closed ward of a psychiatric hospital. Just before our meeting she had tried to commit suicide. She had saved up a couple of months' supply of pills and took about 50 that evening. She wrote a suicide note. She was livid when she woke up the next morning. That should not have happened.

On the ward, just like at home, Laura could really lose her temper. She made the nursing staff pretty standoffish because of her temper. When I entered the ward and asked for Laura, the nurse reacted nervously. She was not uncooperative, but it seemed as if she was scared of her. I was bombarded with questions. 'Does Laura know you are coming?' and 'Do you know it is her birthday?' Next they said to me that they were not sure whether Laura wanted to talk to me. It was noon and she was still asleep. I was taken to a meeting room and left there with a 'hope all goes well' encouragement.

Not long afterwards, Laura entered the room. She had undergone a metamorphosis. Nothing reminded me of the girl I had met a year earlier. Everything about her was black; her clothes, her lipstick and her eye shadow. As opposed to all this black, Laura's face was very white. I knew it was Laura's birthday and had brought a cake. She really appreciated that. During our conversation a bit of colour appeared on Laura's face and her attitude changed from reticent and cautious to spontaneous. Her patient status seemed to disappear. We had a conversation about the subject that occupied us both: her voices.

When talking about her 'upper world' she suddenly said: 'I don't think you should really be able to understand what I am talking about'. For me that was the opening to a reliability test. I answered that, as far as I was concerned, it was not about understanding, but about accepting her experience, how she had lived through it. I did, however, try and draw a comparison with my own experiences. I recognised what she told me about the other world a bit. I had experienced that. Whilst falling asleep, I would go through a tunnel and I would subsequently arrive in a beautiful world with beautiful colours. That world was very real. It was inhabited by people and animals looking like figures painted by Dali; creatures with very thin and long legs which towered high above me. If the colours at the end of the tunnel were dark, I would rather not go inside or I kept on concentrating on the colours until I liked them. Laura reacted to my story by telling me that her other world was only very black and sombre and she also said that she could not step out of it just like that. She had tried once by standing in front of the mirror and slapping herself on the cheek, but that had not worked.

After our discussion, Laura apparently decided to trust me. That became obvious when I got to the part of the interview that dealt with traumas. In the study we looked at whether the children had had traumatic experiences and in order not to miss anything, we had drawn up a list of events which voice hearers themselves had indicated had been the triggers of their voice hearing. Sexual abuse was on this list.

Traumas can inhibit the development of a child. Therefore, in our study we would also look at the development of the child, whether the child developed according to the things that were relevant for its age. Sexuality was one of them. With a 19-year-old girl, you can expect that she will have slept with her boyfriend at some point.

'Do you ever do that?' I asked.

No, I don't do that at all any more. When I was 12 I had an older boyfriend of 23. He would give me weed and then he would let his friends sleep with me. I would be high and disappear into another world. Since that time I have been afraid of sexuality. I felt as if they had made me into a piece of meat. Here on the ward, we have to talk about sexuality in the group. When they start about that, I don't take part. There is a boy here who is in love with me. He has been through things in that area and I trust him. Recently, he spent the night with me, we didn't do anything. I don't want to have anything to do with the others. What I am telling you now, I have never told a soul. I really did not want to talk about it, certainly not to my parents, as they will think that I am a whore.

Suddenly the pieces of the jigsaw fell into place and Laura's high DES score, her upper world, her self-harm, her feeling of guilt, her suspicion, as well as her increasing physical symptoms, became understandable (you cannot suddenly get rid of your sexuality). What an enormous burden Laura has been carrying around for years; something that others did to her.

'I think it was my fault', she says.

'So, your psychiatrists and psychologist really don't know anything about this?'

'No', Laura says, 'and I don't want you to tell them.'

'I think it is important for your treatment.'

'No,' Laura says, 'they don't need to know.'

We talked and talked. Despite all my arguments, Laura was unrelenting and stuck to her 'no'. I was only allowed to tell the psychiatrist about her high DES score and he would simply have to understand it. I did do that, but the psychiatrist did not do anything with the information.

Laura had been hearing more voices in the past year. At this point, she was not just hearing the voice of the ghost, but also the voices of members of her group, her parents and younger sister. The members of the group usually swore, the voice of her father was calming, the voice of her mother advising and the one of her sister swore. Laura heard voices all day long. She started talking to them when she was lying in bed, which made her feel less alone. The voices would take her to another world. Sometimes she was a devil there.

Laura also heard noises. When her head was full of cotton wool, she heard a buzzing tone. Laura saw images of shadows; she thought that other people should be able to see them too (she knew this was not the case). She saw animals being torn apart during which there was a great deal of bloodshed. 'These are horrendous scenes,' Laura said, 'however, I am not really scared of them. When I see these things, I also hear the voices and that does scare me.'

According to Laura the influence of the voices had diminished. She had become more proactive towards the voices as well as the people around her. If the voices disturbed her terribly, she would ask the nursing staff's advice, for example, about her medication. She would not have done that last year. Laura had become more critical of the voices; she had started to check more whether the things they said were indeed true. When she heard the voice of her mother nagging her, she would phone her mother to ask whether it was true that she was thinking bad things about her and she would also ask her to please stop doing that.

Laura did not always carry out the tasks of the voices literally. However, the voices would still appear with all her emotions. She was still scared of the voices. For example, she did not dare go outside on her own any more because of the voices. Laura: 'Sometimes they offer advice; sometimes they say strange things; for example, that other people want to do things to me, or that I am God.'

Last year, the voices made decisions for her, that is why Laura wore so much black, but recently they have started stimulating more independence. Laura said, 'If I want to buy a dress now and I have to choose between two dresses, they say: "Ask your mother, as she has good taste". So that is what I do.'

Laura found that the relationship with the voices had changed. It had become more negative. At first, they would appear less frequently during distractions such as creative therapy or sport, but now that the therapist had doubled the activities of the creative therapy and sport, it no longer worked. It wore her out too much and that is when the voices would appear for longer and longer. Laura could handle an hour of sports, but two hours was too much. Laura had to try and find a balance.

During our third meeting, it turned out that a lot had changed again in the previous year. Laura was at home. The psychiatric hospital had been closed and she had had to choose between a locked ward in another hospital or going home again. She could not face another hospital, so she insisted on going home. Her mother was dreading it, particularly as she found it very difficult to deal with Laura's aggression and her self-harming. Laura had had to seriously negotiate. The result was that she was allowed to go home, under the condition that there would be no extremely violent behaviour and that Laura would take her medication daily. If Laura did not stick to this agreement, she would be admitted again. In return for this, Laura was given her own horse. Laura was crazy about horses. She would do anything to have her own horse. She had already started riding again before the hospital closed. Her mother had seen an advertisement in which the local riding school was looking for a stable helper. Laura, who had been home every weekend, had been hired by the riding school to look after the horses at weekends.

When I arrived by car, Laura was already waiting for me outside. Yet again, I met a different Laura. She was no longer gothic and black, but looked more like the girl I had met for the first time two years earlier. Laura did not want to go in before I had seen her horse in the shed behind the house. After I had admired her horse from top to toe – I am a horse lover too – we went to a cosy kitchen with a long, wooden table where Laura's mother had made me a coffee and joined us.

Laura told me about her daily activities at the riding school. She did not dare go there alone, but that was not a problem as her mother took her. In hospital she had noticed that, with activities, it was all about finding a balance between her energy and her level of exertion. The voices were able to upset the balance. When things were not going well for her, she could cope with less. That did not cause any problems at work, since the owner of the riding school was very understanding. If Laura did not feel well, the riding school owner expected less of her. If the voices were very overwhelming and it was impossible to go on, she would take Laura home. However, that happened very rarely. Laura's passion for horse riding meant that there was a challenge not to let the voices dominate so quickly.

Over the past year, her parents' attitude had changed, particularly her father's. There was more acceptance and concern and both parents talked more about Laura's experiences. Laura had been accepted as a patient. She had been diagnosed as schizophrenic. Both her parents and Laura were in the middle of a grieving process about the fact that Laura was schizophrenic. It was a process that had been explained by the psychiatrist who treated her, where the parents received support too.

At home things went well. Laura's mother told me that she was satisfied about the way things were going at home. So far, Laura had not given any reason to be dissatisfied. She stuck to the agreement. However, at the same time, her mother indicated that she had her heart in her mouth, since she was not sure whether things would stay like this. Laura was in a steady relationship. She showed me a picture of her boyfriend: he was like a kind of Viking, big and muscled with long blond hair. Laura was head-over-heels in love and enjoyed the joys of the world with her new love.

The number of voices had gone down. According to Laura, the voices she heard were the thoughts that other people put into her mind. Laura heard the male voice of the ghost. He would appear about once a week. Further away, she occasionally heard the voices of people she knew, like her little sister, a friend and the voice of her boyfriend. The voices were not just negative anymore. She was able to talk to them a bit.

The voices appeared when Laura was afraid or whenever she felt insecure. At those moments, she did not dare to ride her horse outside. Her mother would always accompany her. However, in the last two weeks there had been a change. Laura wondered whether it would continue. The voices only appeared at night now, when she went to bed.

The voices talked about Laura and other people, about things that Laura preferred not to discuss. Sometimes the voices were nice. If Laura did something well, they would sometimes even pay her a compliment. The voices could also be nasty, as they would force Laura into compulsive actions like holding her breath and walking on ridges. The voices were able to make Laura angry, scared and sad. Laura had to concentrate more because of the horse riding as a result of which she paid less attention to the voices and they had less influence on her life.

Laura was able to hold a conversation with the voices about the other world, but that was happening less often than before. The voices took Laura into consideration and sometimes even admitted that she was right: 'If I think that my father is being a jerk, the voices agree with me, as they know him.' Now that Laura and those around her took her lack of energy into account and thus she was getting less tired, the voices appeared less often. However, the voices had found a new way of forcing Laura to obey their demands. Lately, they had sometimes been threatening, that if Laura did not listen to them, she would lose her mother. Occasionally Laura was very scared of the voices, they could paralyse her with fear.

At our fourth meeting a great deal of progress had been made. The voices had disappeared. Laura had become independent. Last year, she had not dared to ride alone outside, now she was busy with horses outside all day long. She rode the stable's horses for two hours and, after that she rode her own horse, near to her house. Laura's life was as structured as possible. According to Laura, the disappearance of the voices had to do with the fact that she had a set daily routine.

However, when I asked Laura how she saw her future, she went silent and did not know. She had no plans for the future. Laura still did not think life was particularly worthwhile, but she had made a decision. On 18th May, her best friend had committed suicide. She showed me a picture; a beautiful girl with impressive eyes. Laura had decided that, indeed, she wanted to live, so that her friend continued to live through her.

Laura was still considered as a patient by her family and treated accordingly. She was still being treated by a psychiatrist. She would see him for one hour a month. The treatment mainly focused on her medication by checking the drug levels in her blood, and he talked to her parents. Laura did not feel any connection with him at all and therefore, she did not tell him a lot about herself. She did talk about her emotions with the community psychiatric nurse (CPN) who she saw once a month. Unlike how she felt about the psychiatrist, she was enthusiastic about the CPN and trusted him.

Laura still took medication daily. According to her treatment schedule, she would have to continue this for the next five years. Although Laura's mother found that the medication was working, Laura herself did not agree. She saw the medication as a burden; she felt like the medication had changed her into a zombie. Laura once asked me:

'What do you think my voice hearing is related to?'

Laura's mother had joined us at the table. I felt cornered, due to my promise to her not to talk about the trauma. I answered:

'You know very well what I think of this, I told you last year. Don't challenge me. Can I tell your mother?'

'No, I don't want that', Laura said.

To my surprise her mother did not react. I waited and looked at mother and daughter. Nothing happened and I took part in this conspiracy and continued the conversation as if nothing had happened.

Daisy's Story

I met Daisy in 1993 when we were organising the first congress for children hearing voices. Daisy had started hearing voices five years earlier, when she was twelve years old, after her granny had passed away. This granny was the mother of her mother and lived next door. In the first week, all the children of this granny got together at granny's house in order to grieve together. Daisy was not part of this.

During this period Daisy started hearing voices. Initially Daisy only heard one voice; later there were three and sometimes even more. The voices made Daisy feel very insecure. She was looking for information about hearing voices, but could not find what she wanted. When she heard about the children's congress she wanted to take part and even give a talk about her experiences. Daisy is very independent; an independence encouraged by both her parents, such as their support for her wish to give the talk. The talk was prepared by me and she practiced a couple of times. During our practices Daisy had her emotions under control, but when she started talking about the death of her granny in front of a packed auditorium, she burst into tears. Her mother, who was present too, was completely taken by surprise by this. She said that she had thought that Daisy had not been affected by the death of her granny and she had consciously kept Daisy away from all the grieving. During a later contact, her mother told us that she and Daisy had talked about granny's death. The voices disappeared.

I got in touch with Daisy again because of the children's study. She told me that last year she had started hearing voices again. In that period she had been confronted with death twice. During a school trip a girl had a nasty accident, and not long afterwards, the young conductor of the orchestra of which Daisy is an active member died of cancer. The death of the conductor made her very sad. Daisy started hearing voices after his passing away. He was still so young. However, she did feel that she had been able to grieve for him. A memorial service was held, where everyone cried.

Daisy heard voices via her ears. 'It just feels like someone else is shouting something on the inside.' She thought it was someone else, since '... it is not my voice'. She also thought that she sometimes heard music. She smelt funny, chemical smells that other people did not smell. She sometimes felt touches while she was lying in bed awake. When she was a young girl she thought an entire colony of ants was walking on her legs, but now, she thinks, it was her blanket. In the past, Daisy saw balloons that others did not see and once she saw a skeleton in her sister's bedroom, she doesn't have such experiences anymore.

The voices she heard were those of relatives. In the past it was the voice of her granny; now it's her parents' and her sister's voices. In addition, she would sometimes hear many voices: a 'room full'. Her parents' voices tended to be angry, her sister's voice could be nice. Daisy found this strange as she got on well with her parents, but not with her sister. The unfamiliar voices that Daisy heard are those of older people (she thinks around 40 years old).

Daisy usually heard the voices when she was on her own. They could also appear when Daisy was outside, for example, walking to the bus on her way to school, and they would be active all the time. The voices appeared when Daisy was scared, felt guilty, was alone, felt insecure and when she suffered from a lot of stress. The voices intensified her fear and guilty feelings.

The voices were almost exclusively negative and often denigrating. They often told Daisy that she was doing something wrong. The voices set tasks such as that Daisy should not do her homework, since there was no point anyway. They could also tell her to hurt herself, but Daisy didn't listen to that. Very rarely the voices were nice. When she was sad, they could be comforting. They usually talked about Daisy.

The voices made Daisy feel insecure. They could confuse her so much that she could not do her homework well. From time to time they were positive and helped her, by telling her during a school exam that she was able to do well in it. Whenever the voices appeared suddenly, they could sometimes scare Daisy so much that she would panic. Another example of the influence of the voices was that they would shout so loudly at Daisy that she was afraid that other people could hear the voices too. When the voices were shouting at her when she was walking to the bus, Daisy would walk all hunched up, hoping that other people could not hear the voices. Daisy desperately wanted to get rid of the voices, since they were interfering with her daily life.

Daisy had the feeling that she was being controlled, that she was not free. When Daisy felt strong she was in control of the voices. Whenever she felt weak, or suffered from a lot of stress, the voices would control her. Daisy particularly felt like that when the voices were shouting really loudly or when they were holding very devious conversations. She could not conduct a dialogue with the voices because they wouldn't answer. She would sometimes say something to the voices. When she did that, she would talk out loud. Whenever the voices told Daisy to do something, she tried not to do it. However, she did listen.

Daisy thought that voice hearing perhaps had something to do with being able to predict the future or mind-reading. Daisy had this idea that she could read other people's minds. She also thought that she could predict numbers. This regularly happened with a lottery. Daisy knew beforehand which number was going to win. She thought it was a gift and not a illness.

Daisy had an extensive social network. Everybody in her network knew that Daisy was hearing voices. Sometimes she talked about that, when she felt the need for it. She had a girlfriend in whom she confided everything, and she had a boyfriend.

The next time I met Daisy, she was hearing voices in her head. By now she only heard genderless voices of unfamiliar people. Although the voices were never friendly any more, were swearing at her and commented with things like: 'You're not clever; you don't look good', Daisy did not find the voices important any more. She had also started hearing fewer voices.

At secondary school things had not gone well. Daisy largely blamed this on the age difference between her and her classmates. Her birthday was at an awkward time in relation to the beginning of the school year and she had had to repeat a year too. Her classmates were two years younger than her and she did not feel comfortable there. She decided to change schools and she enrolled at a technical college. She was studying civil engineering, but she was the only girl in her year. She liked the school as such, but had to get used to the abundance of men at first. She was concerned that they would not accept her. In the beginning, she felt very unsafe and, during that period, the voices were a lot more active. When Daisy had changed schools, the voices stopped playing such a large part in her life. Daisy no longer paid attention to them that much. At her new school, where nobody knew her, she had made a fresh start.

During the third interview Daisy told me that she was still hearing one voice. She heard a loud, genderless voice of an older person. She had not heard it much. Daisy did not feel safe. She said: 'I don't feel good on the inside.' The reason for this was that she had moved into student digs. As the only girl she was now living in a student house with five boys and one of them was in love with her. She could not avoid contact. Daisy did not have any feelings for the boy who was in love with her. The voice appeared more often.

Although the voice appeared more frequently again and was negative, Daisy did not have anything to do with it. She said: 'I lead my life in a different way now and voices don't fit in.' That is why she wanted to scale down the contact with the voice. She did not want live in the student accommodation any longer, as that was a trigger. Daisy had met a new boyfriend, a boy whose granddad was in a psychiatric hospital. Therefore he had a lot of time for Daisy's problems.

During our fourth meeting, Daisy told us that she was living at home again, like she had planned to do the previous year, since the course at this 'boys' school' and living in a house with just boys caused too much tension. She was studying at home now. The voices had disappeared. She felt safe again. Daisy had a regular inner dialogue now. She said: 'I'm like my mother now.'

Daisy had finished with her boyfriend and felt free again. At home she had renewed her old friendships and therefore she felt less lonely. She did not talk about the voices any more, as she no longer found them of interest. However, she did say that voice hearing was part of her, but at this point in time she did not feel the need to occupy herself with them.

YOUNG PEOPLE
HEARING VOICES

Adults' Section

THE AUTHORS/EDITORS

Sandra Escher, MPhil, PhD, was a science journalist and worked as a senior researcher at the University of Maastricht, focusing on children hearing voices. She is now an Honorary Research Fellow at the Centre for Community Mental Health, Birmingham City University.

Marius Romme, MD, PhD, was Professor of Social Psychiatry at the Medical Faculty of the University of Maastricht (Netherlands) from 1974 to 1999, as well as Consultant Psychiatrist at the Community Mental Health Centre in Maastricht. He is now a Visiting Professor at the Centre for Community Mental Health, Birmingham City University. His research over the past twenty-five years has focused on the voice-hearing experience.

YOUNG PEOPLE
HEARING VOICES

What you need to know
and what you can do

Sandra Escher
&
Marius Romme

First published 2010
New edition 2012

PCCS Books Ltd
Wyastone Business Park
Wyastone Leys
Monmouth
NP25 3SR
UK
Tel + 44 (0)1600 891509
www.pccs-books.co.uk

Young People Hearing Voices: What you need to know and what you can do

A CIP catalogue record for this book is available from the British Library

ISBN 978-1-906254-57-5

Translated from the original by Bettie Goud
Cover designed by Karin Daniels
Printed by Imprint Digital, Exeter, UK

CONTENTS
Adults' Section

PART 3: INFORMATION FOR PARENTS, TEACHERS
AND MENTAL HEALTH PROFESSIONALS

We dedicate this book to the young people
who took part in the study.

Introduction to the Adults' Section

During the course of the study it became increasingly clear to us how little information parents of children* hearing voices were getting and how difficult it was to obtain differentiated information. It also became clear that if, indeed, parents found information, it was almost always based on the assumption that voice hearing was a serious disease. Most parents that we met could not accept that. That assumption is only logical if you believe that voice hearing means that your child is crazy and probably suffers from schizophrenia.

The consequence was that they could not accept the voice hearing of their children either. They did not dare to talk about it; they were scared of it. Most parents we met started searching for information and that is a good thing. We noticed that the children of those parents who dared to search and go their own way were doing better. This book is for these parents. It contains a lot of information; information which can help you develop your own ideas about hearing voices. Dealing with a child who hears voices is like going through a process in which the voices are accepted and the child will be supported based on the acceptance. It is a 'searching together'.

In this section of the book we have also included some information from and about alternative therapists. This is because we found that parents were more enthusiastic about alternative therapists than psychiatrists. Often they would search and find advice from alternative therapists out of dissatisfaction with orthodox psychiatry, particularly when they were rather lavish with diagnoses and drugs. However, they

---

* Throughout this section where the word 'children' is used this also includes young people or adolescents.

would then get stuck. Therapists in the regular healthcare sector often refuse any contact with alternative therapists or forbid parents to consult them and subsequently assume that they, indeed, do not do this. We often saw this happening in our study too. Some parents would go and see an alternative therapist, but not tell their regular therapist. However, we also saw conventional therapists who had the courage to work together with alternative therapists, where the alternative therapists looked after the voice hearing and the psychotherapists dealt with the other problems. Therefore we have also included information about alternative therapies.

In this section you will find stories from a few mothers. Some also talk about their contact with me (Sandra). This is not the reason why I have included these stories, but I have done so to give you an example of how normalising the experience can give some peace of mind and open the way to accepting voices and wanting to know more.

Parents and child, you need to look for what suits you and, at the beginning of the process, you need to be as well-informed as possible. Please do not forget that voice hearing is not a disease as such, but it can make you ill if you do not learn how to deal with the voices (and any underlying problems).

1

The History of Hearing Voices

This chapter does not pretend to be able to give a total overview of the historical course of voice hearing. A whole book might do it credit and several authors have already written on the subject for different purposes and from different points of reference (Slade & Bentall, 1988; Thomas, 1997; Watson, 1998). On the other hand, ignoring the history would not be helpful for understanding why this kind of research, for example, the adult study on hearing voices and this children's study, was done.

Hearing voices has been reported in the histories of the ancient civilisations of Egypt, Rome, Babylon, Tibet and Greece (Watson, 1998). In these earliest societies positive voices were commonly reported. It was believed that at certain sacred sites it was possible to obtain advice and guidance on important decisions from the voice of a god. In later times, it was more common that these divine messages were mediated through appointed priests or priestesses The earliest well-known voice hearer is Socrates (469–399 BC). Although he reported hearing the voice of a daemon, he valued the voice positively.

The first hypothesis about hallucinations came from Aristotle (384–322 BC) who did not relate them to his own experience. According to Aristotle, voices were produced by the same mechanism which normally produces hallucinations during sleep, the mechanism of dreaming (Feinberg, 1970).

Experiences of voice hearing are often mentioned in a religious context. Significantly, people identified as founders of religious movements reported hearing voices: Jesus (Christianity); Mohammed (Islam); George Fox (Quakers) and Joseph Smith (Mormons). Both in

the old and new testaments, Moses, Jesus, the apostle Paul and Maria all declared having heard voices. It is known that the Abbess Hildegard of Bingen, the saints Teresa of Avila and Francis of Assisi, and the protestant Luther heard voices (Watson, 1998). Probably the most well-known voice hearer is Joan of Arc (1412–1431) who perhaps gives the earliest example of a voice hearer where political events had a great influence in the way people looked at the her experiences. She was openly known by her troops to be guided by voices when she took them into battle to free France from the English. However, when she was captured she was accused of witchcraft due to the voices. In fact, her trial was the political debate about who would own the French crown.

The first noticeable change toward hearing voices might be seen in relation to the development of individualisation as part of the evolving European cultural movement of the Renaissance. It was a time regarded as the emancipation of mankind from the powers that dominated its existence: that of the clergy and the state. Across much of Europe during the Middle Ages, political power was in the hands of the Roman Catholic Church, as Church and State operated as one body. The Church functioned as the prime controller of knowledge and the development of independent thought represented by individualism threatened the power of the Church.

As early as the fourteenth century one can find the first traces of the Renaissance and individualisation in the work of Dante (1265–1321) who was a poet, statesman and a philosopher. In his text *Monarchia* (Winkler Prins, 2002; Perler in Routledge 2000), Dante proposed that the aim of civilisation was the gathering together of human potential to obtain peace and freedom. Dante held revolutionary ideas where he proposed that the individual, state and church should have separate roles, where the role of state and church should provide guidance rather than control. In the fifteenth and sixteenth centuries the developing influence of the Renaissance was so strong that it included all facets of daily life and all types of art, such as architecture, painting, sculpture, music, copper-plating, tapestry and glass blowing. It also influenced views on, and thereby treatment of, ill people (Thomas, 1997).

Until the early Renaissance, theories of disease were still grounded in astrology and alchemy (Thomas, 1997). Medical changes became

the consequence of an apparently harmless revival and interest in Classical Greece. This interest was stimulated by the interest in the human body where, for example, the artist Leonardo da Vinci published a series of anatomical sketches, which in turn influenced the Belgian anatomist Vesalius, who studied medicine in Paris. Vesalius was taught in the traditions of anatomy unchanged since Galen (around the second century BC), who in his work extended the theories of Hypocrates. To learn more about anatomy, Vesalius undertook dissection, a very risky business as the Church had forbidden this; the Roman Catholic Church regarding the structure and function of the human body as God-given, sacred and not for men's eyes (Thomas, 1997). Vesalius' actions and observations thus challenged ideas sacred to Christianity; for example, the belief that women had one more rib than men and that the heart was the centre of the mind.

Many others challenged the established views of the Church. Copernicus calculated that the sun, not the Earth, lay at the centre of the solar system, a view at that time that was seen as heretical. Inventions of the telescope, thermometer, barometer and microscope provided the means by which the early scientist philosophers could delve ever more deeply into material properties of the natural world (Thomas, 1997: 153). The Church perceived the development of science as a threat, as the acquiring of knowledge through scientific exploration effectively made God and the Church redundant. Therefore the Church sought means to retain control, and across Europe it greatly expanded the system of inquisition to detect heretics. The Inquisition started around 1184 in Rome where it was legislated by Pope Lucius III and it finally stopped in 1772 in France:

> In order to defend Christendom against Satanic influences, Pope Innocent VIII ordered in 1489 the publication of the book *Malleus Malefircarum* (The Hammer of the Witches). This book set the conditions for the burning of people who were suspected of witchcraft or possession by demons. (Slade & Bentall, 1988: 6)

It was a brutal system run by monks who were given wide-ranging powers such that their actions were not accountable to the local bishops. When heretics were detected, they were brought to trial according to the

Catholic laws. The Inquisition was thus much feared and, at such a time, reporting hallucinations was clearly a danger to one's life.

Teresa of Avila (1515–1582), who was an abbess, was able to save a number of visionary nuns from the machinations of the Inquisition by introducing concepts of 'sickness' and 'lack of responsibility'. She explained that certain 'natural causes' were capable of explaining the visitations, namely (a) melancholy; (b) a weak imagination; or (c) drowsiness, sleep, or sleep-like states (Slade & Bentall, 1988: 6). Thus it was Avila who developed the first medical concept concerning hallucinations born out of a political need. Positive reports of voices thus disappeared, but whilst this did not mean that the experience no longer occurred, a strong cultural taboo was created.

The second historical influence on the contemporary attitude towards hearing voices is the cultural development in the period of 'Enlightenment'. This movement started around the sixteenth century, where it is related to the era of British 'Glorious Revolution' and the end of the French Revolution (Winkler Prins, 2002). This period is also called 'the episode of philosophy', a time when people were challenged to use their minds, challenging beliefs that a human being could not use his reason as he was bound by superstition, prejudice and the powers that maintained these. The new optimistic view was that, through reason, one could separate what is natural and what is unnatural (Thomas, 1997).

Influential to the Enlightenment movement was the French philosopher Descartes (1596–1650), with his 'Cartesian' system of thought regarded as the foundations for the science of psychology (Thomas, 1997). His famous phrase 'I think and therefore I am' introduced 'dualism' that conceptualised the separation of body and mind.

> Our understanding of the world is located in internal experiences, in the mind of the individual. The twin peaks of Cartesian thought, mind/body, that opened the way for the materialistic study of human behaviour, and the belief in the foundation of knowledge through the experience of the individual, has had a potent effect in shaping psychological thought. In particular, it has stimulated scientific approaches aimed at understanding the

internal mechanisms of minds, and their relationship to brain. The problem is that it has led to neglect of the relationship between the individual and other(s), for as Russell observed, morals and ethics, those aspects of philosophy that understand the values that govern our individual and social relationships, had little or no place in Cartesian thought. (Thomas, 1997: 157–8)

In the centuries that followed, this scientific approach became the dominant culture with all the consequences. The tools of science are objectivity assured by the condition that what is accepted as knowledge must be produced by methods and, thus, results that are replicable. By separating the body and mind, Descartes created the possibility to study the mind as an object, separate from the body and from the environment, as if there is no interaction, no relation whatsoever (Thomas, 1997: 2003).

With the development of science, terminology developed as well. In relation to experiences such as hearing voices, the term 'hallucinations' was for the first time introduced by Lavater in 1572 (Slade & Bentall, 1988). He based it on a translation of Galen's conception of madness as 'a disturbance of bodily humours'.

> The word 'hallucinations' is an anglicised version of the Latin 'allucinatio' (wandering of the mind, idle talk). The term was used to refer to a variety of strange noises, omens and apparitions. (Slade & Bentall, 1988: 7)

The French physician Esquirol (1832) conceptualised hallucinations in an attempt to distinguish between 'insane' and 'sane' hallucinations. He differentiated these extraordinary experiences into illusions and hallucinations.

> People who suffer from hallucinations are dreamers while they are awake. Hallucinations are 'memory recalls without the intervention of senses'. (Slade & Bentall, 1988: 8)

The insane were mistaken by the nature and cause of their present sensation. Illusions, on the other hand, were seen as situations where:

> ... the sensibility of the nervous extremities are excited; the senses
> are active, the present impressions call into action the reaction of
> the brain. (Slade & Bentall, 1988: 8)

The distinction between 'insane' and 'sane' was strongly debated. Esquirol described the insane as 'mistaken by the cause of the present sensation', while, in 1855, the French Société Medico-Psychologique distinguished insanity in relation to the inability to control the experience. Both arguments still play a role in the contemporary debates.

However, insanity did not restrict itself to an individual illness but existed within a social construct.

> It was Esquirol and his teacher Pinel who rejected the view of
> mental illness as a self-acting entity, independent and alienated
> from the community of people that produced it. To the contrary,
> they argued, how much the mental patient and the normal had in
> common. In attempting to refute the notion that the mental
> patient was globally disturbed, possessed, they attempted to
> differentiate precise symptom pictures. In what they called 'folie
> raisonnante' a patient might at times have a different perception
> of reality than his examiner, but in many other aspects he might
> be reasonable. It is by some lamentable misinterpretation of
> history that Esquirol is now reported in the textbooks to deserve
> credit for the modern mystifying use of the term hallucinations.
> (Rabkin, 1970: 115)

According to Rabkin (1970), it was not Esquirol's idea to diagnose a person as an individual without reason.

> By defining the two terms, Esquirol's main purpose was to point
> to the rest of the patient's behaviour and circumstances, behaviour
> which was rational. This is usually not mentioned. (Rabkin, 1970:
> 116)

CATEGORISATION INTO ILLNESS ENTITIES AND THE CONSEQUENCES

In this part we will first briefly explain the development of illness categories and of diagnosis in order to argue why it has become inadequate in relation to voice hearing.

In the second half of the nineteenth century and in the first half of the twentieth century, mental illness was often still considered in terms of the interaction between environment and individual. Under the influence of Freud's philosophy, Adolf Meyer attempted to integrate Freudian theory into the practice of clinical psychiatry:

> Meyer's approach to understanding mental illness was normalising, in that he regarded it as an understandable reaction to a set of life experiences. His approach was significant in the importance that it attached to the person in understanding mental illness. His approach focused on persons not patients. (Thomas, 1997: 148)

At the same time a small but powerful group in Germany criticised this social approach (Kreapelin, Bleuler). They found working with the psychosocial model unscientific, believing that it would fail to generate any meaningful research in the field of mental illness. They, instead, wanted to refine the pathological concept that attempted to explain mental illnesses from within a biological or genetic frame of reference.

> Kreapelin (1856–1915) developed a classification system for mental illnesses. His first modest overview was published in 1883 as *Compendium der Psychiatrie*, followed in 1887 by a second edition, *Psychiatrie: Ein Lehrbuch für Studierende und Ärzte*.
>
> Once Kreapelin had decided to devise a classification of his own, it took him a decade to develop the dementia praecox concept.
>
> It was not until years later that it was transformed into psychiatry's prime nosological concept at a time when his general classification was being expanded as well. (Blom, 2003: 53)

> It was in 1911 that the first monograph on schizophrenia appeared. It was written by Eugen Bleuler who had introduced the term

> schizophrenia three years before, replacing Kreapelin's concept
> of dementia praecox. (Blom, 2003: 42)

Expressions of mental illness were no longer seen as understandable reactions to a set of life experiences, but as expressions of an illness entity, an underlying illness of the functioning of the brain. The influence of this line of understanding mental illness is predominant in medical faculties nowadays. Textbooks structure the first medical ideas of medical students – the doctors-to-be. This kind of thinking is the first step toward learning to use diagnosis on the basis of symptoms, categorised into illness entities without aetiological knowledge of these symptoms.

However, with this approach, Kreapelin and, with him, clinical psychiatry had little regard for what the symptoms (of the illness) the patients were alleged to be suffering from might mean for them (Zilborg & Henry, 1941). However Kreapelin's system became a great success.

Slade and Bentall formulated their criticism:

> The development of specified illnesses has all kinds of consequences which might be considered negative.
>
> Firstly the medical model has led to the study of syndromes rather than symptoms. Most research into abnormal behaviour over the last 50 years or more has taken diagnostic categories such as 'schizophrenia' or 'depression' as independent variables.
>
> Secondly the view that hallucinations are medical phenomena has led to a relative lack of interest in them by psychologists. (Slade & Bentall, 1988: 9)

Slade and Bentall are right in their criticism, but in the first half of the last century psychiatrists felt in need of a diagnostic system to establish whether certain symptoms were so characteristic that they make the diagnosis for a certain illness. Therefore, the psychiatrist Schneider (1959) developed a refined scale to describe verbal hallucinations which he thought were specific for schizophrenia. He distinguished: '... hearing voices that speak your thoughts aloud; hearing two or more voices talking about you (in the third person, referring to you as "he" or "she"); hearing one or more voices carrying on a running conversation in which

your actions or thoughts are commented on.' Schneider put forward that one of the characteristics of his distinguishing factors was indicative for the presence of the illness of schizophrenia.

However, the existence of this kind of reality is hypothetical. As Mary Boyle states:

> What is perhaps most remarkable about their work (Kreapelin, Bleuler, Schneider) is that in spite of aligning themselves to a scientific framework, not one of them presented a single piece of data relevant to their assumption that they were justified in introducing and using the concept of dementia praecox and schizophrenia. (Boyle, 1990: 75)

In our own study (Romme, 1996), no clear differentiation between characteristics of verbal hallucinations were found, experienced in patients diagnosed with schizophrenia, with dissociative disorder or in the non-patients (people with no psychiatric illness when assessed with the CIDI (Robertson, 1988)).

Whilst it is clear that criticism can be levelled at diagnostic systems, the recognition of disease entities had much to offer clinicians, encapsulating a desire to work scientifically, culminating in the development of the *Diagnostic and Statistical Manual* (DSM) of the American Psychiatric Association.

> It was a victory for biological psychiatry over the psychosocial movement and psychoanalysis in particular. Its detailed prescription of criteria for the diagnosis of mental illness has had international implications. It proved a firm basis for diagnosis which generated a new impetus in biological research. (Thomas, 1997: 149)

However the development of the DSM was not according to prevailing scientific standards, as it was not essentially based on research. The DSM was created from a questionnaire sent to 2000 American psychiatrists asking their opinions concerning mental illness, with the consequence being that no social circumstances were taken into account.

Criticism on this classification system started more openly at the end of the 1980s, resulting, amongst others, in the publication of a number of seminal texts; Richard Bentall's (1990) *Reconstructing Schizophrenia*, Mary Boyle's (1990) *Schizophrenia: A scientific delusion?*, Phil Thomas' (1997) *The Dialectics of Schizophrenia* and Dirk-Jan Blom's (2003) *Deconstructing Schizophrenia*.

Criticism has also grown out of daily practice, questioning the utility of the diagnosis, so that today the diagnosis of schizophrenia has enormously diminished in credibility amongst many practitioners (van Os & McKenna, 2003). In the Maudsley Discussion Paper (No. 12) Jim van Os express the following concern:

> The DSM definition is severely biased towards non-affective symptomatology. The reason for this discrepancy is likely to be related to the need of medical practitioners to convince of illnesses as clearly separable disease entities, based on the old Kreapelinian distinction between poor-outcome schizophrenia and good-outcome affective illness. (van Os & McKenna, 2003)

There is also clearly an argument for why this DSM classification system is inadequate for voice hearers, as it does not incorporate the significance of the social context. In the Maastricht research, which looks for a relationship between the voices and the life history, great care was taken to clarify the onset of the voices and any traumatic events at that specific time. About 70 per cent of the voice hearing in adults began after events, including death of a family member, divorce, moving house, losing a job, sexual abuse (Romme & Escher, 1989). The events occurred in social circumstances, and happened to people beyond their control. The voices often tell about circumstances that created an overwhelming experience of powerlessness. Voices are messengers of the problem or problems of the voice hearer. In any diagnostic system, including the DSM, the social context and the content of the voices need to be included and not excluded in order to understand the experience and the need of the voice hearer. Instead of moving forwards, the medical profession seems to have lost this social context, something that was taken on board in the beginning of the last century. In the search for scientific objectivity, psychiatry seems to have lost the patient.

As the clinician Rabkin formulates it:

> It is my contention that Esquirol's worst fears have been realized, that his term has achieved the opposite of his intention: namely that the psychiatrist as alienist, as he used to be called, has created a set of alienating ideas or ideologies, prominent among which is hallucinations, which he mistakes for the real world of behaviour as one can mistake the image in the mirror for the veridical perception. By using these myths to alienate his patients in space he has alienated himself in a much more profound fashion. (Rabkin, 1970: 116)

SUMMARISING THE DIAGNOSTIC SYSTEM IN RELATION TO HALLUCINATIONS

The DSM is a categorisation system with no scientific validity. It is a classification system not a diagnostic system because it does not include aetiological factors. In the DSM manual the psychosis is described as:

> The term psychotic has historically received a number of different definitions, none of which has achieved universal acceptance. The narrowest definition of psychotic is restricted to delusions or prominent hallucinations, with the hallucinations occurring in the absence of insight into their pathological nature. A slightly less restrictive definition would include prominent hallucinations that the individual realizes are hallucinatory experiences. Broader still is a definition that also includes other positive symptoms of Schizophrenia (i.e., disorganised speech, grossly disorganised or catatonic behaviour). (DSM-IV: 273)

This reduces the scope on hallucinations and is not open for the reality which we observed in our research: that hallucinations have a meaning and should not be alienated from the person.

CHILDREN

The discussion so far has followed the history of voice hearing and the development of the categorisation and diagnosis for adults. Whilst the beginning of contemporary psychiatry can be situated in the middle of the eighteenth century, child psychiatry did not develop until the beginning of the twentieth century. There are two influential factors that stimulated its origin (Hart de Ruyter & Kamp, 1973; Timimi, 2002), both generated from socio-cultural developments. At the end of the nineteenth/beginning of the twentieth century, juridical authorities no longer wanted to judge deviant and criminal behaviour of children only as punishable cases, instead seeking psychological causes in the development of the child and looked for causal influences in the environment. The reason for this change of policy was that it created a possibility to educate and treat those children, as well setting a line for prevention. In this way one might create preventive measures to avert asocial behaviour developing into delinquent behaviour. The second factor in the development of child psychiatry was the rise of the child guidance clinics during the 1930s, founded in the United States and later promoted in Europe.

In the beginning, child psychiatry was the domain of neurologists, with the development of child guidance clinic care extending this to the multi-disciplinary team. It thus took political power from within the medical profession to establish the specialism of child psychiatry (Hart de Ruyter, 1973).

Concerning hallucinations, there is relatively little known about children and hallucinations. There is some literature including Freud and Bleuler (Kemph, 1987) relating auditory hallucinations to childhood. However, their observations were not based on research on children. One of the earliest studies undertaken with children with hallucinations was by Bender and Lipkowitz (1940), who stated that it was difficult to distinguish between the normal and the pathological experience. However, Despert (1948) had a different opinion, asserting that a three-year-old child is able to distinguish reality from fantasy and thus does not have genuine hallucinations. According to Despert, genuine hallucinations are, in Freud's concept, formulated as regression to gratify infantile wishes, passing beyond the testing of reality. She

therefore concluded that they are simply not present in very young normal children, stating that children from ten years of age have similar hallucinations to those of psychotic adults.

Kemph (1987) argued that the only difference between adult and child hallucinations is that they are simpler and lack organisation and systematisation. Kemph studied 331 psychotic children between six and 15 years of age and found no hallucination in children under eight years of age. The group from 8–11 years of age had a significantly higher incidence (68 per cent) of hallucinations than the older children. He suggests that this might be because young children have more primitive defences and less firmly developed ego functions such as 'reality testing' and a tendency to think in terms of concrete objects and actions.

Other researchers like Bender, Jaffe, Lucianowicz and Esman (in Rothstein, 1981) gave more attention to the role that psychodynamics might have in the case of hallucinations. They tried to find a relation between hallucinations and social cultural variables. Specific background variables (but not as the only cause) necessary for the presence of the experience like social class, race, gender, deprivation, poverty and/or isolation from prime carers.

In the past and present literature there are different opinions, which contradict each other about the age at which children are able to experience hallucinations and about the cause. In the last 15 years, children have become more the focus of attention or – one could say – become more popular in research. In clinical studies of children and adolescents, auditory hallucinations may occur in the context of a variety of psychiatric states such as schizophrenia (Bettes & Walker, 1987; Green et al., 1992; Galdos & van Os, 1995; Galdos et al., 1993), anxiety and depression (Garralda, 1984; Ryan et al., 1987; Chambers et al., 1982), migraine (Schreier, 1998), trauma, dissociation processes and reactive psychoses (Altman et al., 1997; Famularo et al., 1992; Putnam & Peterson, 1994) and deprivation (Bender, 1970).

Nearly all studies concern selected clinical samples, and a small number of children. Long-term follow-up of such groups suggests variable outcomes, reflecting the heterogeneity of the subject selection procedures in the different studies (Garralda,1984; Del Beccaro et al., 1988).

Slowly interest is developing in the experience in a non-clinical setting. The first study of non-patients was that of Yeates, who in a

study of three subjects described hallucinations as a reaction to grieving (Yeates & Bernnard, 1988). Altman et al. (1997) and Schreier (1998) report on 'not treated' children; they continue to use the word 'non-psychotic' children, still relating it to an illness.

However, no short-term sequential follow-ups of children with hallucinations have been conducted to study the course of these experiences and the possible factors that influence their short-term course. Little is known about the course of hearing voices and the outcome in relation to the pathways through care. This children's study is aimed at this gap in knowledge.

Although research shows that hearing voices is present in patients and non-patients, contemporary daily practice of child psychiatrists mostly follows the general psychiatric approach in adults. The key word is diagnosis. Hearing voices might be an early symptom of psychosis and those children are seen as at risk of developing schizophrenia later in life. As clinicians work with diagnosis or are expected to use diagnosis for organisational reasons, this might force a more medical approach than is helpful (Timimi, 2002). Child psychiatry research has come to rely too heavily on medical-model-inspired methods as the gold standard.

One consequence is that medication, for example Ritalin, has become ever more popular and is promoted as the best treatment (Timimi, 2002). This approach might make the child dependent on the medical system and does not stimulate and activate the self-healing capacities of the child. It takes power away instead of stimulating it: 'You are ill, you might have schizophrenia' is not the best start to overcoming the problems and to receiving support.

However, it is not only the medication that can be problematic, but also the rules set by the therapist. Children and parents may be forbidden to talk about the voices as, in line with the clinical opinion, talking about the voices reinforces engagement with the hallucinations. To see the voices primarily within an illness construct may well be the first step on a path that becomes defined by social disadvantage and stigma, manifesting as discouragement, or even exclusion, from educational opportunities, obtaining particular types of employment or accessing some types of insurance, acquiring a driving licence or the mortgage for a house. These are consequences that might not be

seen when the child needs care where, according to standard procedures, a diagnosis with a psychiatric illness such as schizophrenia is given.

Timimi (2002) warns about this medicalisation of childhood and thus the outcome of this children's study is directly relevant to Timimi's conclusions. As child psychiatry is a relatively young profession, the outcomes of the study can provide a significant contribution to existing ideas and practices, with the potential to develop a new direction. Professional input should not be the only option the child is given. In adult psychiatry the influence of the user perspective has become more important (Kleinman, 1988; Coleman, 1996; Read & Renolds, 1996; Boevink & Escher, 2001). Child psychiatry has to engage in these debates about cultural, political and social contexts (Timimi, 2002).

2

Current Theoretical Explanations
within Mental Healthcare

> Any percept-like experience which (a) occurs in the absence of
> an appropriate stimulus, (b) has the full force or impact of the
> corresponding actual (real) perception, and (c) is not amenable
> to direct and voluntary control of the experiencer. (Slade &
> Bentall, 1985: 23)

This is a definition of an auditory hallucination.[1] Within the mental
health system there are many different theoretical explanations for
the phenomenon of hearing voices, the most common of which have
been developed from the disciplines of psychiatry and psychology.

PSYCHIATRY

The medical discipline of psychiatry can be differentiated into clinical,
social and biological theories. These differentiations have developed
over time and will be discussed further in Chapter 1 as this
differentiation has had a great impact on the way hearing voices is
regarded. Clinical and biological psychiatry have become the dominant
perspectives within psychiatry, postulating that, as with physical
diseases, psychiatric illnesses are caused by biological or genetic
impairments. Over the last 50 years extensive research has been
undertaken in an attempt to prove this. Social psychiatry has never
been recognised as an autonomous science, though it has a clear
theoretical framework which embraces the interaction between the

---

1. As this chapter explains theoretical concepts in which hearing voices is called auditory
hallucination, I have used this term here, although in my work in never use this term as
it alienates the voice hearer from what he/she experiences.

person and his/her environment. Social psychiatry became established in the 1970s, but has since lost ground in its development as a science and is particularly challenged about its scientific methods and evidence. However, as psychiatry can be likened to a small society with political parties (see Chapter 1), it might also be said that social psychiatry did not have the political organisation to represent it in the political battlefield of science and research funding. Currently in The Netherlands social psychiatry continues to be practised in community mental health services, having the opportunity to operate independently of those hospital-based services influenced by clinical and biological psychiatric theories.

Current clinical, biological and social psychiatric practice uses different theoretical explanations concerning auditory hallucinations. Those different starting points have significant consequences for treatment. These basic theoretical differences within psychiatry apply equally to adults and children.

Clinical psychiatry

In clinical psychiatry hearing voices with the characteristics of an auditory hallucination is seen as a symptom of an illness. The explanation of the voice hearer for this experience is mostly interpreted as a delusion. In the DSM-IV (APA, 1994) (diagnostic categories are further discussed in Chapter 1: 9ff), a broadly accepted categorisation system for psychiatric illnesses, auditory hallucinations are interpreted as a psychotic symptom and only mentioned as a symptom of schizophrenia. However, the scientific validity of the diagnosis of schizophrenia is quite doubtful (see Chapter 1). It is lacking in construct as well as content validity (Bentall, 1990; Boyle, 1990; Blom, 2003; van Os & McKenna, 2003).

Biological psychiatry

Biological psychiatric research on hallucinations is looking for causes in the brain. Deformations were found in several parts of its structure (Barta et al., 1990; Culberg & Nybäck, 1992; Foster & Caplan, 1994) as well as several dysfunctional areas (Green & Preston, 1981; Musalek et al., 1989; Cleghorn et al., 1992). However, these findings are unsatisfactory in explaining the cause of the voice hearing experience.

The findings of these studies were also not repeated (Thomas, 1997). In some studies a relationship between auditory hallucinations and activity in the brain centre was found (McQuire et al., 1993), however this is not seen as a causal but as a simultaneity, simply meaning that when someone experiences the hallucination there is activity in the brain, possibly indicating an inner speech phenomenon.

Social psychiatry
In social psychiatry, illness behaviour (symptoms and experiences) is regarded as a reaction to overwhelming social problems and personal interactions, with which the person has not been able to cope. Hearing voices is seen as a reaction with a context. Social psychiatry relates to four levels of influence interacting with each other; organic, individual, social and societal (Romme et al., 1981). Theoretically it refers to the general systems theory (Bertalanffy, 1950; Miller, 1967).

Throughout our previous research we demonstrated that hearing voices functions as a reaction pattern when someone is not coping with social problems. It leads to all sorts of secondary reactions mimicking in some patients the clinical complex of schizophrenia. The relation between hearing voices and sexual abuse is already well established in patients with a diagnosis of dissociative disorder (Ensink, 1993; Herman, 1992). This relationship has not been demonstrated with schizophrenia patients, though this is currently being proposed as a study by Mike Smith at UCE, Birmingham.

PSYCHOLOGY

Whilst in psychiatry voices are most commonly accepted as the symptom of an illness; in psychology hallucinations are in principle not seen as an illness but as a deficit and are related to reality testing (Bentall & Slade, 1985, Slade & Bentall, 1988). Theoretically, psychology has more to offer for voice hearers as it is aiming at possibilities of growth and the ability of learning to cope with the voices. As psychology is a very diverse field, this section will restrict itself to the more established developmental theories that are used in psychology in relation to the development of voice hearing and also are used in research.

Developmental theories
Reality testing

In children, auditory hallucinations are often related to fantasy or to imaginary friends. Fantasy that is perceived as real such as fantasy friends are a quite normal experience for young children. For example, Singer (1973) found, in a study with 141 three- and four-year-old children, that 65 per cent of them reported having playmates; playmates as fantasy made real. Piaget provides evidence that children below the age of eight years often report dreams as being real (Piaget, 1974). As a child grows older he/she should be able to distinguish between fantasy and reality, though in the literature there are significant differences in the age that this transition occurs, and Despert (1948) argues that children with an average intelligence could distinguish fantasies and reality at the age of three years; Harris et al. (1991) argue that children between four and six years of age do not always feel certain that an imaginary monster cannot become real. Foley et al. (1983) see the age of six as a turning point; Piaget (1974) believed it to be eight years and Golomb and Galasso (1995) state that children at the age of four are able to distinguish between fantasy and reality, even when they experience overpowering emotions. Coren and Saldingen (quoted in Rothstein, 1981) propose that the ability to distinguish between fantasy and reality develops after the child goes to school.

In the above literature there is agreement to the fact that, at a certain moment in the development of children, imaginary friends ought to disappear. Children whose imaginary friends don't disappear might develop a lifelong inability. However, Taylor et al., (1993) disagree, arguing that children with imaginary friends possess a richer fantasy world that allows them cognitive as well as emotional advantages.

This inability to distinguish between fantasy and reality is explained by the hypothesis that very young children think that all information comes from the outside world. Their own thoughts are interpreted as coming from outside and are understood as the reality. Within this context auditory hallucinations are accounted for as their own thoughts projected outside of themselves.

Slade and Bentall (1988) and Bentall and Slade (1985) focused their early research on reality testing and found a significant relationship

between auditory hallucinations and poor reality testing. Slade proposed that because people with auditory hallucination are not able to test their first perception accurately to the original stimulus, they would hear seemingly unrelated words (Slade, 1976). Bentall and Slade (1985) found that people experiencing auditory hallucinations are more easily convinced of the presence of stimuli, even though they might not be present.

Theory of mind

Bentall and Slade's work is grounded on a 'theory of mind'. The theory of mind refers to human's ability to form accurate impressions of other people's intentions and the way they feel about others. Three stages are mentioned:

1. the ability to understand that one has a mind of one's own;
2. to understand that others have a mind;
3. using that knowledge to make assumptions: understanding that what you think might be false; also to distinguish between fantasy and reality.

Before the age of six, children understand little about the influence of mental processes on reality. From six years onwards, children know that knowledge might come from participation of the mind and that is how they are able to draw conclusions (Flavell et al., 1993). In itself, the theory of mind does not explain auditory hallucinations, but this theory is of influence in developmental theories.

Self-monitoring

The process of self-monitoring developed from the theory of mind, which also distinguishes steps. The first step in self-monitoring is to formulate the intention. The next step is to establish a plan of action in order to complete the task. In this step feedback mechanisms are fully integrated. However, in order to initiate and complete a task, a person must be able to monitor what is going on and this, in itself, stresses the importance of self-awareness. In order to be able to do self-monitoring, an individual must have gone through the three stages of the theory of mind outlined above successfully.

The theory of self-monitoring was developed by Frith (1992) who based it on earlier work of Hoffman (1986), who relates auditory hallucinations to an inability to communicate effectively. In his studies Frith relates the development of monitoring to auditory hallucinations. He reasons that, if the mechanism of self-monitoring breaks down, this might explain the positive and negative symptoms of schizophrenia, one of them being hallucinations. He argues that, if a person fails to recognise his thoughts relating to his observations of others, he interprets them as either inserted into his head by others, or he might hear the thought about his observation of others as a voice (Thomas, 1997: 50). Hallucinations occur when preconscious hypotheses about the nature of the stimulus fail to be filtered out, so that too much information intrudes into consciousness (Bentall, 1990: 116).

Development of inner speech

Communication and language seem to be central issues in relation to auditory hallucinations. A theory that underpins auditory hallucinations in this way is that of the theory of inner speech. The idea here is that inner speech might be interpreted as coming from a source in the outside world. In general, young children seem to relate inner sources more often than an outer source. Flavell et al. (1993) state that it is not because children prefer external sources, but that they do this if the information they receive is too diverse and too complex. If this happens, they are not able to distinguish between internal or external sources.

Again, in the literature there are diverse opinions about the development of inner speech and the ages related to this development. Some researchers do not think it is possible for young children to experience inner speech, whilst others think they could have it. Two established scientists who hold these opposite opinions are Piaget and Vygotski; Paiget being French and Vygotski a Russian.

According to Piaget cognitions provide language. The development of speech would follow:

inner speech ⟶ egocentric speech ⟶ social speech

Between 18 and 24 months children begin to think in symbols, which appears from the basic structures of the sensory-motorial thinking. Because language is stipulated by the mind, the early speech, as well as the thinking, is egocentric. When a child grows older, the realisation that other people have thoughts too originates the real dialogue (Cole & Cole, 1989). This would mean that children are able to experience auditory hallucinations at a very early age.

Vygotski reasons the other way around. For Vygotski, philosophically influenced by Marxist theory, processes of the mind always occur within a social and cultural context. He proposes that the development of thinking and speech are separate processes till the child is two years of age. Language is the key to the development of thinking and, when children develop language, mental processes change. Thinking becomes restructured into speech.

Vygotski reasoned the development of speech as follows:

$$\text{social speech} \longrightarrow \text{egocentric speech} \longrightarrow \text{inner speech}$$

In the first phase, social speech, the child learns from adults the contents of words. In the second phase, the child will use words to give direction to its behaviour; the child starts talking out loud to itself, just like the adult who gives instructions (Burritt, 1991). At the age of three there is no difference between social and egocentric speech, and by the time the child goes to school, egocentric speech disappears when inner speech develops.

When applied to auditory hallucination, according to Piaget, it is natural if young children experience auditory hallucinations. In older children it is, therefore, related to errors in their development. According to Vygotski, children are not able to experience auditory hallucinations until the age that they go to school and experience inner speech, when they might interpret inner speech as coming from a source in the outside world. Following Vygotski's reasoning, the content of the inner speech would be influenced by the outside world, by social and cultural influences. Research confirms the idea that inner speech plays a role in the process of coping with hallucinations, although the evidence does not make clear in what way (Leudar & Thomas, 2000). In the children's study we saw that 33 children developed inner speech

during the research period. Of those children, 32 had lost their voices (see Chapter 6).

Summary

Hearing voices is, within clinical and biological psychiatry, seen as a symptom of an illness. In social psychiatry voices are seen as a reaction to problems relating to social circumstances. In psychology voices are interpreted as a deficit relating to a stage in the development and information processing as in reality testing.

The consequences of the theoretical framework for the voice hearer and his/her treatment are enormous. In clinical and biological psychiatry, medication is seen as the most adequate treatment. Social psychiatry focuses at the relation between the voices and problems and the treatment will include coping as well as working through the underlying difficulties. In psychology the focus of treatment will be aimed at development; for example, learning to cope with the voices.

PSYCHOANALYSIS

In this section I will refer to psychoanalysis because in our adult research it became clear that a number of voice hearers used their voices as a 'defence mechanism' towards certain threatening emotions. Psychoanalysis originally conceptualised the idea that individuals develop psychological coping mechanisms in response to the experience of overwhelming emotions. Therefore, it can be argued that the psychoanalytic theory of defence mechanisms is an important body of knowledge in understanding the process of coping with voices. In psychoanalytic theory the symptom (experience and behaviour) comes instead of an emotion. In this sense the psychoanalytic theory has greatly improved our understanding of psychiatric symptoms. However, in the literature, hearing voices is seldom described as a defence mechanism because psychotic symptoms have mostly been explained otherwise. An exception is the work of Pruett (1984) who relates it to the area of young children. Based on a single case history, he proposes that voices might be explained as a primitive defence mechanism of young children who, at an early age, still rely on magical and primitive solutions to cope with trauma.

In the psychoanalytic literature auditory hallucinations are described as resulting from either direct symbolic repetitions of psychical traumas, or as criticism of the superego, or as regression to a lower perceptual level of thinking (Heilbrun et al., 1983). Several studies have been undertaken to explore these three causal explanations:

1. Auditory hallucination might reflect physical trauma. The hallucinations are a conversion symptom and they often consist of reproductions of memories from events from the past with emotional value (Andrade & Srinath, 1986); for example, loss of a loved one (Yeates & Bernnard, 1988). Also Wenar (1994) relates them to trauma. Putman proposes that some memories are isolated in the conscious and return as hallucinations (Bernstein & Putman, 1986).

2. Auditory hallucination might be related to functions of the superego. Rothstein proposes that hallucinations form an externalised conscious (Rothstein, 1981). Yeates and Bernnard state that hallucinations are developed because of incomplete internalisation of the superego (Yeates & Bernnard, 1988). According to Despert (1948) they might appear when a child is very frightened and experiences an inner conflict.

3. Auditory hallucination might be related to regression to a more primitive stage. Implicit to this psychoanalytic vision is that in certain phases in his life a child is vulnerable for auditory hallucinations. Quoting Freud: 'Hallucinations are a form of regression to a more primitive phase in the development.' Quoting Despert (1948): 'Auditory hallucinations originate by regression of the child to more primitive behaviour from which burst instinctual desires.' Quoting Yeates and Bernnard (1988): 'It is cognitive regression ... Children hallucinate deceased family members ... This implicates restoring the deceased.'

Summary

In the psychoanalytic idea auditory hallucinations might be seen in relation to trauma, the development of the superego or regression to a more primitive phase. These different functions have different consequences for the way auditory hallucinations are defined and

should be treated. However, all three tendencies relate to auditory hallucinations as an individual reaction and relating it to the individual does not acknowledge the social interaction. As is shown in research, hallucinations are often related to trauma caused by others (Romme & Escher, 1989; Ensink, 1993). Although psychoanalysis is helpful in understanding coping with emotions it tends to neglect the social influences of trauma and social interactions especially in situations where psychotic experiences are found. It thereby isolates the voice hearer from their experiences and social realities.

OTHER PSYCHODYNAMIC THEORIES

The literature discussed so far stresses the pathological aspects of voice hearing. In some psychodynamic theories, hearing voices is seen as normal, so that voices might be heard by people who are functioning well in daily life. In these theories, auditory hallucinations are explained as a form of coping mechanism or a tool, in order to cope with life-events. The adaptive value of voices is stressed (Heilbrun et al., 1983). Although psychodynamic theories originate from the work of Freud and auditory hallucinations are seen as individual experiences, they are also seen in relation to environmental influences.

This section has been added for two reasons. In our research on adults (Romme & Escher, 1989, 1993, 2000) and for this study, one of the aims was to look for a relation between voices and a person's life history. In about 70 per cent we found a wide range of traumatic experiences in relation to the onset of the voices and most were due to environmental influences.

The second reason for adding this section is that we often found that voices can be seen as messengers (Romme & Escher, 1989 , 1993, 2000). In psychodynamic theory, the content of the voices, what the voices say, is acknowledged as significant. Negative voices are not only seen as pathological, but negative and aggressive voices might have an adaptive function through the aggressive satisfaction they give, or they might symbolise the nature of the relationship with others.

There are several studies that relate voices as a way of coping with trauma. Boon et al. (1990) postulate hallucinations as a form of

dissociation in situations of trauma, such as grief. They see voices as split-off parts of the mind that might be experienced as not-me. Those voices might have a protective task as they split off the traumatic experiences (Boon & van de Hart, 1990).

There is also a tendency to relate auditory hallucinations to coping with object relations. Rothstein (1981) proposes that voices might protect children in their relations with others. Bender (1970) points out that hallucinations occur with children who show psychodynamic problems. The hallucinations are helpful in shaping interpersonal relations within deprived children. Flavell et al. (1993) relate hallucinations to deprivation or separation from parents, resulting from a retarded cognitive functioning. Kospodoulus et al. (1987), on the other hand, describe voices as a form of dissociation of the self, resulting from isolation and lack of affective support in periods of stress. According to this theory, people who hallucinate try to maintain reality in spite of difficult circumstances. According to Yeates and Bernnard (1988) who published three case histories of children hearing voices as a reaction to grief, voices might compensate for the absence of important emotional others. Simonds (1975) proposes that hallucinations are an attempt to externalise internal stress like anxiety, depression and guilt. Research findings from Linville (1987) show that auditory hallucinations might form a buffer for the negative effects of stressful events on body and mind.

Summary

Psychodynamic theories do not always relate auditory hallucinations to pathology, but explain them as a normal reaction to influences, caused by circumstances created in the environment; grief, deprivation, stress and problematic relationships with others. In psychodynamic theories voices are explained as a tool or mechanism to cope with these life events. The voices are seen as metaphors and as messengers. Therapy based on psychodynamic theories is less dogmatic than in psychoanalysis.

COGNITIVE PSYCHOLOGY

> The cognitive science arose largely as a revolt against the simple reductionist approach of behaviourism which until than had dominated psychology. In its simplest form, behaviourism states that all human actions can be understood in terms of learning and theories of association. In contrast, cognitive science emphasises the role that thinking processes play in our behaviour. It places 'mind' firmly in the domain of psychology. (Thomas, 1997: 46)

Cognitive psychology is a relatively young branch of psychology. Its origins are based in the therapeutic setting with the founder of cognitive behavioural therapy, Aaron Beck (1952). He developed a method for coping with depression that is now used for auditory hallucinations as well. Beck proposed that the fundamental problem of the individual was that he/she developed a negative set of beliefs, or 'cognitions', about themselves. These beliefs have a powerful influence and are not supported by facts. Later research by Richard Bentall gave an enormous impulse to implant Beck's model in relation to auditory hallucinations (Beck, 1952). Cognitive psychological research on hallucinations is centred on abilities or rather disabilities concerning language. Again there are very diverse findings in this field of research.

Auditory hallucinations might be caused by intellectual deficits such as in the domain of command of the language (Heilbrun & Blum; Johnson & Miller; Miller, Johnson & Richmond; quoted in Bentall, 1990). Garralda reports of a deficit in the domain of the reading abilities (Garralda, 1984). Other research describes a relation between cognitive schemata and information processing. Brand found that people diagnosed with schizophrenia do not have access to schema that rule auditory hallucinations (Brand, 1986). Rund found that people diagnosed with schizophrenia construct in an unknown manner, not existing stimuli (Rund, 1986). However, most research has been conducted on patients – and mostly on patients with the diagnosis of schizophrenia.

Other studies relate auditory hallucinations to mental images. Green and Preston found in their research that people diagnosed with schizophrenia experience whispered speech as auditory hallucinations (Green & Preston, 1981). Heilbrun found that psychiatric patients could

relatively poorly recognize words, meaning and grammar of their own thoughts when spoken out loud. This poor knowledge of their own thoughts could be the reason why these people attribute these to an external source (Heilbrun et al., 1983). Heilbrun also proposed that patients with auditory hallucinations might have a lesser preference to auditive images (thoughts in words) than to visualized images (Heilbrun et al., 1983).

Again, in this area there are contradictory findings. Seitz and Molholm concluded that lack of auditory imagination is an essential condition to experience auditory hallucinations (quoted by Slade in 1976). Mintz and Alpert (1972) found that schizophrenic patients with a history of auditory hallucinations reported a significant number of strong auditive images compared to a control group of schizophrenic non-hallucinators. Slade (1976) reported that psychotic patients generally reported stronger mental images than a control group. It is worth making two critical notes; first, that the contradictory findings do not give a consistent idea about the origin of hallucinations, and second; that most of the research was done with patient populations.

In the last twenty years, research has shown that people who are hindered by the voices often develop their own coping strategies (Falloon & Talbot, 1981; Breier & Strauss, 1983; Cohen & Berk, 1985; Tarrier, 1987; Romme & Escher, 1989; Romme et al., 1992). People can learn to react to their voices in order to learn to understand and cope with them (Chadwick & Birchwood, 1994; Birchwood et al., 2000).

In the recent decades a lot of research has been undertaken to develop cognitive therapy for psychosis by a great number of British psychologists. Slade, Bentall, Haddock, Birchwood, Turkington, Kingdom, Chadwick and Tarrier have all developed different methods to influence the beliefs people hold concerning the voices through therapy.

Summary
Cognitive behavioural therapy and research has shown that voice hearers are able to learn to cope with the voices and that there are more or less effective ways of coping. Voice hearers are supported and encouraged to talk about their voices and this, in itself, reduces the anxiety about the voices.

SUMMARISING THIS CHAPTER

In psychiatry and psychology there are a number of explanations on which therapy for people who hear voices is based. In psychiatry, clinical and biological psychiatry restrict hearing voices to an individual illness from which people should be cured. However, research does not provide evidence that there is only one single explanation for voice hearing. Looking at contemporary research and the accounts that voice hearers give, there appear to be other possible explanations. For example, in recent literature, trauma is related to the onset of both hearing voices (70 per cent) and psychosis (Thomas, 1997; Ensink, 1993). A trauma is not an isolated individual event, but must be seen from a social and societal context. In these cases, social psychiatry offers a much broader frame of reference than clinical and biological psychiatry, as it interprets voices as a reaction to problems and using a systemic theoretical base, with influences on four levels (organic, individual, social and societal).

In social psychiatry, illness behaviour (symptoms and experiences) is regarded as a reaction to overwhelming social problems and personal interactions with which the person has not been able to cope. Hearing voices is seen as a reaction with a context.

In psychology a different perspective is taken. Hearing voices is related to a deficit in developmental areas and therapy aims at learning to cope with this deficit.

However, one must not forget that professional theories are guidelines for professionals in order to make sense of the experience and to establish a therapeutic plan. These theories do not necessarily relate to how voice hearers experience what is happening to them. As Ron Coleman, a voice hearer, has stated: 'Psychiatry takes away my experience, moulds it into their model and then hands it back in a way unrecognisable to me.' In the research on adults and children it has became apparent that the therapeutic relationship (see Chapter 6) was more important than the theory and people experienced a better relationship to a therapist who used theories they felt related to their experience.

3

Non-medical Explanations
of Voice Hearing

If voice hearing should not be considered a disease, what indeed could it be instead? In the medical model a great deal has been written about voice hearing, but outside of it too. By just reading the Bible, you will discover that it is a book full of voice hearers – Jesus, Moses and Abraham all heard voices. The Bible explains voice hearing based on religion. There are also the mystics, people who are searching for enlightenment, who hear voices. Searching for enlightenment is not necessarily linked to religion, but to spirituality. For instance, Buddhists describe voice hearing as a phase in the process of spiritual development. This phase precedes the phase in which the monk is so enlightened that he lifts himself off the ground. In the Catholic Church's history, we can also find a number of mystics who heard voices, for example, John of the Cross and Teresa of Avila.

Shamans are known for searching for enlightenment in order to achieve greater wisdom. The process of spiritual development is consciously begun. You can only become a shaman after a period of fasting and mortification, during which you will undergo special experiences like voice hearing. Moreover, there are also famous people who heard voices such as Joan of Arc who was told to fight the English. Socrates heard the voice of a demon, the psychiatrist Jung heard voices, as did Ghandi and Churchill. It shows that if you hear voices you are in good company. It would be going too far to discuss the spiritual development in religion and shamanism in greater depth in this book, since this does not relate to children. However, the progression of their development is crucial.

This chapter deals with only a limited number of explanation models, since we noticed that explanations weren't very important for children, particularly those younger than 12, but it was important for their parents. Explanation and a language for the voices are essential elements in dealing with the voice hearing experience.

Back to our study. What explanations did the children have for their voices?

- 16% thought that their experience was linked to religion;
- 20% thought that they were ghosts/phantoms;
- 18% thought that the voices were linked to another world;
- 20% had another explanation;
- 39% thought it was a special gift, like a paranormal experience.

VOICES AS A SPECIAL GIFT

Most children thought that voice hearing was linked to a paranormal gift. When children state that their voices are linked to a paranormal gift, two basic principles are important.

Someone can think that he/she has a paranormal gift, but they need to remain critical. Not every experience which you may think is a paranormal gift is actually one in reality and, even more importantly, not everyone has a paranormal gift. Whether someone has a paranormal gift can be tested.

Paranormal experiences only take place under certain conditions. In order for it to be a paranormal experience, there needs to be an emotional relationship with the person you can hear and there needs to be a change in the level of consciousness. If you think you are having a paranormal experience, you can check this yourself by asking the actual person that you think you are hearing whether this is true or not; whether that person, indeed, thought or said what you were hearing. Learning to check whether it is true is good, since it will make you less suspicious. If you hear a voice which says that the person you are talking to may look very sweet, but in the meantime thinks that you are stupid and you believe it is a paranormal experience and therefore true, it will then be difficult to remain nice to that person.

You will start to mistrust that person. Who knows what else he thinks of you?

There are quite a few young people who attribute one or more of their voices to this kind of experience. Voice hearers are very sensitive people who can easily pick up other people's emotions, but do not recognise these to be someone else's and assume that these are their own emotions. A voice hearer may, for instance, hear the voices of the neighbours who can be heard through a thin separating wall and, thus, believe that these are his voices. It could also be that a voice hearer reads other people's emotions on their faces, but does not realise that he is doing it. These emotions can start having a voice. When you realise that you are doing that, you need to learn to shut yourself off from outside influences.

Almost 40 per cent of the young people who hear voices said that they had this gift. There were quite a few who learned to deal with their gift through a psychic. In the second year of our study, one of the boys had even started his own psychic practice. He was coached by his aunt, who had the same gift. Most did not feel this need. One boy said: 'Working with my gift may happen at a later stage, when I'm ready for it.'

A paranormal gift can cause confusion when things are not going too well for the voice hearer, such as problems at school or at home. He gets little sleep or does not sleep well. If that happens the voices become stronger and the voice hearer suffers more from the voices. In such a situation a voice hearer is more prone to thinking that other people are talking about him. It is, therefore, more complicated to find out what is the matter, for example, since embarrassment could play an important role.

I know a female voice hearer who, whenever we had had a conversation about her voices, would hear my voice at night saying all kinds of nasty things about her. At first she believed that I really did say such things. She would then find it difficult to say something nice to me the next time we were in contact with each other. After a while, she learned to ask me whether the things that she thought I said had, indeed, been said by me. It was a great relief to her to discover that the voice had fooled her. The problem of the voice had still not been solved, but it was not made worse. Later on in the book, I will discuss this further.

The disadvantage of this belief is that the voice hearer can get the idea that all kinds of people can influence their mind or at least get into their head.

HEARING VOICES AS A RELIGIOUS EXPERIENCE

Amongst adult voice hearers there are many who think that voice hearing is linked to religion, however, these were not people who believed in a specific church or who went to church. Sixteen per cent of the young people saw a link between religion and the voices. An eight-year-old girl told me she was hearing the voices of two Jesuses. One was a good one, the other a bad one.

Religion has several objectives. For centuries it steered the daily lives of millions of people. The church took over a great deal of responsibility from its believers. It decided what was good and bad. With the diminishing interest in the institutional church, I do not mean the building, the dialogue between good and bad has not disappeared. There has been a shift from feeling connected and a sense of togetherness to individual, spiritual development. Not only did we lose the connection to others, we also had to start deciding for ourselves what was good and bad; which information we regard as 'true' and practise in our lives. Particularly when people have problems due to circumstances that cause stress, or disease, loss and death, they will look to spirituality in order to get in touch with a greater entity. That, in turn, gives a feeling of connection. It could be that the religious explanation fits with the need for spiritual development. Every religion has come into being as a result of a mystic experience. It could also be that the religious explanation fits with your attitude to life and your vocabulary. Almost every voice hearer feels the need to verbalise his experience in order to understand what he is experiencing; an explanation accepted by other people, feeding the need to feel togetherness. Within the religious explanation death has a place and, therefore, fear of death can be discussed. This was something that a number of voice hearers really needed. Young children are, after all, occupied with death. They can bombard you with questions at a time when they are having any experience of death at all. Almost a third of the children started hearing voices after the

death of a grandparent, another relative or a friend.

Religion and spirituality are also very difficult to translate into numbers; they are not a science. You cannot really prove it. You cannot overwhelm someone with figures or show impressive brain scans. It is about experiences that other people recognise. Therefore, you need to find people with similar experiences who can guide you. The disadvantage of this view is that if nobody around you still believes in God or life after death, it will not be easy to talk about it. If you can't talk about it, you, as a voice hearer, will isolate yourself too much.

VOICE HEARING AS A NORMAL EXPERIENCE

For parents, the fact that a child hears voices is, in itself, a reason to believe that it is a disease. Only eight per cent of children hear voices; most without being really disturbed by it. Voice hearing is a normal experience but does not happen to everybody. In our Western culture we are scared of it.

In Africa, for instance, it is a common belief that the spirits of the deceased will hang around on Earth for a while and that they have something to say. People who can communicate with spirits are, as medicine men, greatly appreciated within their community. Indonesia and Surinam also have a culture in which spirits of the deceased are in contact with the village doctors. Moreover, there are millions of people in India who think that voice hearing is linked to events in a previous life. This way of thinking is called reincarnation. Reincarnation is rebirth. It is assumed that the soul lives a lot longer than a human life. After the person dies, the soul goes back to a kind of waiting room from where it will go to a new body.

Almost 40 per cent of the children think that voices are linked to ghosts or phantoms or that they come from another world. If these children explain their voices as ghosts, phantoms or coming from another world and they are not afraid of this, please do not make your child scared because of your own fear (as a non-voice hearer); accept the explanation and find a language to talk about it together. We do not live in Africa, but there are plenty of children's books with stories in which children are in contact with ghosts, phantoms or beings from another planet.

The disadvantage of this view is that people in our Western society remain scared of voices and, therefore, they cannot accept them. If a child wants to talk about his own experience and his parent does not accept his voices, the child will alienate himself from his own experience and cannot then learn to deal with it. A child can deduce from your choice of language whether you accept him and also whether you can listen to his/her experience as he/she experiences it. A good introduction to this is the book *Listening to Children* by the American psychologist Dr Thomas Gordon.

I hope that through this explanation of the various models I have been able to make it clear that if you are looking for help because of your child's voices, you need to show a real interest in the origin of the voices. You need to accept that voice hearing is a personal experience which varies from one person to the next. What works for one person does not necessarily work for the other. What I am trying to say here is that you and your child need to develop your own ways of thinking in order to deal with the experiences. You cannot go to a doctor and say: 'Here I am with my child/my problems; please solve them, I'll wait here while you do that.' A doctor can support, ask questions, encourage, help you learn to deal with your fears. It is your child who needs to be able to deal with his voices. As a parent you can provide important support. The voices can be a pain, a real pain and have a lot of influence on family life. Your doctor cannot solve the problem. If your child is prescribed medication, you need tosee if it does what it is supposed to. If it does not work write this down before you go and see the doctor and also write down why you think it does not work. In the first year of our study only three children believed that their voices were due to a disease; most of them found it difficult, but believed it to be normal. Today most of the children from the study have recovered and quite a few have forgotten about the voices altogether.

SUMMARY

In our study 80 children told us about their experiences and all of the 80 experiences were different. Certainly not every child had a clear explanation for the voices. It was often a bit of this and a bit of that Furthermore, during the course of the study explanations changed.

Children were not that interested in these explanations, but their parents were.

Voice hearing is an experience which does not happen to everyone, but it is normal. Disease develops as a reaction; when there is no control over the voices and the relationship with the voices is bad. Since it is an unusual experience, you will look for an explanation. An explanation can help in finding a language for that experience, to understand it better and to communicate with others about it.

Most children came up with explanations outside the medical model. Almost 40 thought that it was a paranormal experience, but a socially acceptable experience. One of the mothers said, 'It is something I can talk about to the neighbours or the teacher at school.' At the end of the study children and parents described that accepting voices, the experience and the possible explanation of the voice hearer was important to them. Only by accepting voices can recovery begin. If the voices are not accepted, conflict continues, and no one learns from their experiences.

If you have not developed an understanding of the problem, you can occupy yourself a lot with the voices. However, you must realise that there is more to life than voice hearing, although it may not seem that way at first. For almost all of the children, the voices were the central point of focus during the first interview and this changed completely by the fourth interview. Some could not even imagine that they had ever heard voices. For most of them it was a relief to notice that other things had become more important, like friendships, sports and going to school.

That does not mean to say that all problems had suddenly been solved, but they were looked at differently now. Most young people had learned to deal with the emotions linked to their problems in a better way.

4

Young People Who Hear Voices:
The role of psychiatric treatment
Professor Sami Timimi

Fourteen-year-old Raheena was brought to see me by her parents after her school asked for an urgent appointment due to noticing a dramatic change in her behaviour. She had become withdrawn, at times laughing inappropriately, and at other times bursting into tears for no apparent reason. Raheena tells me that she's been hearing (and sometimes seeing) a 'spirit' who comes into her body and then comes out again and passes out through the walls of their house.

Ten-year-old Charlotte was brought to see me by her father who has been given a diagnosis of schizophrenia and has been hearing voices since his adolescence. Charlotte has started self-harming by sometimes scratching herself with a sharp object. She discloses that she sometimes hears a male voice 'in her head' that tells her to do this. Her father is worried that she may be developing his 'illness'.

Seventeen-year-old Chris lives with his grandparents. For the past few weeks he has become increasingly withdrawn, looks preoccupied, has stopped attending college and is not sleeping well. He explains that he hears voices 'screaming' at him in his head that remind him of his mother and father when they used to 'beat' him as a child. He is terrified by this experience.

Sixteen-year-old Samantha is doing well at school, has a good circle of friends, but has recently started superficially scratching her upper arm. Her mother brings her to see me after becoming concerned when Samantha told her that she hears a voice that repeats the phrase 'nobody loves you' to her.

Fifteen-year-old Gavin is arrested by the police after assaulting a pupil at his school. The police notice he is behaving 'bizarrely' and

believes that people are trying poison him and is suspicious of professionals who come to see him. He refuses to talk to me initially. After I guess correctly that he is scared that he is going 'mad', he cries and tells me about voices he's been hearing telling him people are after him because he is a 'worthless gay'.

Seventeen-year-old Ellie has long-standing conflicts with her easy-going parents. She explains that she has been hearing a variety of voices since she was about five years old. She does not experience these voices as threatening or unwelcome. In fact, she finds her inner world with its conversations and exchanges of ideas with these 'voices' more interesting than the 'outer' world.

Hearing voices isn't a uniform experience. There isn't just one interpretation that you can place on their significance. Nor, for that matter, is there just one remedy for those who experience voices that they find distressing. Some young people have many voices for many years; some have a single voice for a few weeks. Some feel threatened and controlled by these 'voices', others less so and others still experience them as welcome or even friendly. Some feel compelled to follow any instructions the voices give them or take seriously the voices personal comments towards them, others are more able to ignore them or challenge them.

For many it is a signal that they are in a state of distress. How I, as a professional, then respond to that distress could have a significant influence on what happens in the coming weeks, months and even years of their lives. In this chapter I will discuss some of the scientific evidence that should be taken into account when professionals consider how to respond to young people presenting with experiences such as the ones listed above.

PSYCHOSIS AND THE MEDICAL MODEL

According to current mainstream orthodoxy, the experience of hearing voices should be viewed as a 'symptom' and the task of the psychiatrist is to consider this, together with an account of other 'symptoms' and history of the 'illness', in order to arrive at an accurate diagnosis of what condition (mental illness) has caused this symptom to manifest itself. For psychiatry, hearing voices (which is technically described as

'auditory hallucinations') is invariably considered as an 'abnormal' experience. Although there is some acknowledgement that extreme stress (for example in bereavement) or physical illness can cause temporary states where a person may experience auditory hallucinations, this symptom is usually considered to be one that points toward a serious mental illness (such as schizophrenia) and a state of 'psychosis' (where the person is considered to have 'lost touch' with reality through such 'abnormal' experiences). Psychotic illnesses are generally viewed by mainstream psychiatry as having been caused by biochemical imbalances in the person's brain and therefore need to be treated with medication (to correct these assumed biochemical imbalances).

However, empirical support for this narrow 'medicalised' view of such experiences is limited and there is much evidence to suggest that adhering to such a view and trying to persuade the sufferer to adopt this view may have an unintended negative impact on that person.

For example, researchers have long been aware of the perplexing finding in cross-cultural studies that those diagnosed as having 'schizophrenia' (widely considered the most serious and often chronic psychotic illness that 'causes' auditory hallucinations) who are in developing countries appear to fare better over time than those living in industrialised nations. Research, including that carried out by the World Health Organisation over the course of 30 years and starting in the early 1970s, shows that patients outside the United States and Europe had significantly lower relapse rates. It seems that the regions of the world with the most resources to devote to mental illness – the best technology, medicines, and the best-financed academic and private research institutions – had the most troubled and socially marginalised patients (Hopper et al., 2007). For these sufferers, the impact of Western psychiatric technologies seemed to be minimal compared to psychological and social factors such as family support, community cohesion and tolerance for behaviours and experiences considered a sign of 'illness' and 'dangerousness' in the West.

Read and colleagues' (2006) comprehensive review of the literature on stigma and schizophrenia, found an increase in biological causal beliefs across Western countries in recent years, suggesting that the idea that experiences such as hearing voices are being caused by

'abnormal' brain chemistry is gaining hold in Western societies. However, biological attributions for psychosis were overwhelmingly associated with negative public attitudes. This appears particularly to be the case for the diagnosis of schizophrenia. For example, Angermeyer and Matschinger (2005) subjected two representative population surveys of public attitudes to psychiatric patients conducted in Germany in 1990 and 2001 to a trend analysis. Over the period of the study an increase in public acceptance of biomedical explanations of psychosis was associated with a public desire for an increased distance from people with schizophrenia.

This 'medical model' of psychosis not only increases public stigma, but also contributes to patients internalising an explanatory model that can hinder their recovery. For example, it has been found that the presence of 'insight' (in psychiatric terms, meaning accepting the medical model of having a brain illness) in schizophrenia lowers self-esteem, leads to despair and hopelessness and also predicts higher levels of depression and risk of suicide attempts four years later (Crumlish et al., 2005). Hasson-Ohayon and colleagues (2006) found that the presence of this sort of 'insight' was negatively correlated with emotional wellbeing, economic satisfaction and vocational status. The conclusion we may draw from this body of research is that the empowerment of people with psychotic symptoms and helping them reduce their internalised sense of stigma are more important than helping them find insight (in medical terms meaning accepting they have an 'illness') into their problems (Warner, 2010).

Thus it seems that part of the reason why the outcome is better for those who develop a psychotic episode in the developing world is less stigma, and that it is the medicalising approach that is more likely to produce stigma and the sense of alienation, disability and shame. Trying to find out how this may sometimes work, the anthropologist Juli McGruder spent a number of years in Zanzibar, Tanzania studying the families of those diagnosed with schizophrenia. Though the population is predominantly Muslim, Swahili spirit-possession beliefs are still prevalent and commonly evoked to explain the actions of those who violate social norms. McGruder found that, far from being stigmatising, these beliefs served certain useful functions. The beliefs prescribed a variety of socially accepted interventions and ministrations

that kept the ill person bound to the family and kinship group. McGruder saw this approach in many small acts of kindness, watching family members use saffron paste to write phrases from the Koran on the rims of drinking bowls so the ill person could literally imbibe the holy words. The spirit-possession beliefs had other unexpected benefits: this way of viewing the mental distress allowed the person with schizophrenia a cleaner bill of health when their symptoms improved or stopped. An ill individual enjoying a time of relative mental health could, even if just temporarily, retake his or her responsibilities in the kinship group. Since the illness was seen as the work of outside forces, it was understood as an affliction for the sufferer but not as an identity inscribed through unalterable internal factors such as his or her genes (Watters, 2009).

OTHER PERSPECTIVES ON HEARING VOICES

In psychiatry and psychology there are also other explanations for the experience of psychosis and hearing voices. As mentioned above, the dominant view in mainstream psychiatry attributes hearing voices to an individual illness for which people should be given medication. However, other views are available, even if they occupy a less powerful influence than the dominant psychiatric one. Research has highlighted a strong connection between trauma and the experience of both hearing voices and psychosis (Romme & Escher, 1989; Thomas, 1997; Read et al., 2004). In this model the experience is regarded as a reaction to overwhelming social and personal problems. Other theories relate hearing voices to a deficit in certain developmental tasks that have not been adequately achieved; but perhaps more interesting are those that have developed outside of professional circles, particularly the reflections of those who hear voices themselves about the meaning and function of these experiences. Sadly this perspective is frequently ignored by professional discourse and institutions.

As Ron Coleman, a voice hearer, argues, psychiatry takes his experience, moulds it into their model and then hands it back to him in a form that is unrecognisable to him (Coleman, 1999). Much of this 'user' literature tries to reframe the task of 'therapy' or healing into one that takes seriously the content of the voices, trying to understand

its potential personal meanings (for instance, particular traumatic experiences) and finding pathways to 'recovery' through self-help. This may not necessarily involve getting rid of the voices, but instead learning how to get on with one's life, whether the voices remain or not (Romme et al., 2009).

Voice hearing can also be framed as a 'normal' experience. Research has confirmed that the experience of hearing voices is not always associated with dysfunction or a clinically diagnosable psychiatric disorder. Marius Romme (1996) found no clear differentiation between characteristics of verbal hallucinations experienced in patients diagnosed with schizophrenia, with dissociative disorder or in the non-patients. Indeed, in many cultures, voice hearing is not viewed so pathologically. Not only do many cultures believe that it is normal that the spirits of the deceased continue to communicate long after their death but, in addition, those who can communicate with spirits (who often experience what we psychiatrists would class as auditory hallucinations) are often viewed as having 'gifts' that give them qualities that are greatly appreciated within their community and provide them with social status (such as becoming a shaman or traditional healer).

HEARING VOICES IN CHILDREN AND YOUNG PEOPLE

The experience of 'hearing voices' in children and adolescents has been found to occur in the context of a variety of psychiatric states, such as schizophrenia, anxiety, depression, migraine, trauma, dissociation processes and reactive psychoses (Escher et al., 2002). A population-based epidemiological study found that the prevalence of at least sometimes experiencing hallucinatory phenomena in children was eight per cent, of which only a third qualified for a formal psychiatric diagnosis (McGee et al., 2000). In another study involving 761 children, self-reported psychotic symptoms at age 11 years increased the odds for psychotic illness at age 26 years by about 16 times, but the actual number who went on to develop a psychotic disorder was very small (Poulton et al., 2000). For the majority of children experiencing hallucinations in the general population, therefore, these experiences appear to be non-pathological. A small group, however, may develop

persistent symptoms and subsequent psychotic disorder in adult life. In another study, a group of 80 children (with a mean age of about 13 years) who were hearing voices were followed up over a period of three years. It was found that over this period about 60 per cent stopped experiencing voice hearing. Those who perceived the experiences to influence their behaviour and feelings and had more negative appraisals of them, were more likely to be 'patients' requiring or seeking further professional help (Escher et al., 2002).

TREATMENT WITH MEDICATION

There is a long history in psychiatry of exorbitant claims being made for a variety of practices from insulin comas to radical brain surgery such as lobotomy. Each new 'advance' brought with it enthusiastic claims of 'miracle' cures, which, over time, when subjected to rigorous objective research, were shown not to be as effective as first claimed with risks having been unduly minimised. In recent decades, waves of optimism about 'curing' and 'treating' mental illness through modern psychopharmacology has popularised the use of psycho-pharmaceuticals, changing the prescribing habits of doctors and the health-seeking behaviour of patients. Sadly, closer scrutiny of the scientific evidence reveals that the new age of the mass use of psychopharmaceuticals is more the result of good marketing than of good science; through a confluence in the interests of neo-liberal politics, the profit motive of pharmaceutical companies, and the 'self-interest' of psychiatrists (Moncrieff, 2008a). Closer scrutiny of the science shows that, as in previous eras, physical treatments for psychiatric disorders and claims for the curative properties of psychopharmaceuticals have been exaggerated and their dangers minimised (Whitaker, 2002; Moncrieff, 2008b).

The treatment of children with psychiatric drugs is even more contentious than that of adults as many of the drugs now being used on children are meant for, and have only been researched in, adults. In a context in which no objective tests exist to verify the 'diseases' being diagnosed, pharmaceutical companies realise that a bigger market for their product can be created by 'disease promotion' (Moynihan et al., 2002). Here the task of the pharmaceutical company becomes that of

convincing the medical profession and the public that young people's emotional and behavioural problems are the result of under-diagnosed and under-treated 'brain' disorders which, of course, sets the context for their products to be marketed as 'treatments' for these alleged physical disorders. They do this by a variety of methods including sponsoring or producing material for doctors' waiting rooms that alert the medical and lay community to the existence of these conditions, producing 'educational' material for parents and teachers and funding parent support/campaigning groups.

However, the problem is not just that of the profit motive of pharmaceutical companies, as the problem of professional identity, while making child psychiatry vulnerable to manipulation, must also be owned by the profession. Child psychiatry should sit at the confluence of many different systems of knowledge: medical, psychological, social, paediatric, anthropological, cultural and so on. The move towards favouring biological models and physical treatments has been attractive to sections of the profession that wish to carve out a clearer territory that bolsters a more 'doctor-like' image of what they do, rather than the more diffuse, hard-to-define role a more complex approach that spans several disciplinary territories provides (Timimi, 2008).

The main form of medication used by doctors to control or 'treat' auditory hallucinations and/or a psychotic illness are so-called 'anti-psychotics' (I say so-called, as categorising medication as 'anti-psychotic' implies a specificity in 'treating' psychosis; a specificity which these drugs most certainly do not posses). I will address the problems of using anti-psychotics with children and adolescents by referring to two publications on this subject that are widely considered in the medical community as important.

The first publication doesn't deal directly with the use of anti-psychotics for psychotic states or experiences, but looks at the use of anti-psychotics in those diagnosed with 'autism'. I discuss this because it reveals the importance of looking beyond what 'opinion leaders' in the field claim. In this article, 'opinion leaders' Susan Morgan and Eric Taylor (2007) take an apparently moderate stance suggesting that anti-psychotic drugs should not be used indiscriminately in children with autism but should be reserved for those with more 'serious' behaviour

problems. This apparent moderate position still contains within it justification for using anti-psychotic medication for 'aggressive' behaviours in those diagnosed with autism. They state that: 'We consider off label use [of anti-psychotics] is justified when other approaches fail or are unfeasible' (Morgan & Taylor, 2007: 1069). This effectively leaves the door open for the continued increase in the use of anti-psychotics as the reading doctor is left to wonder what other approaches to use and for how long before deciding they have failed. Furthermore, unfeasibility of other approaches is near universal as the increasing popularity of the diagnosis of autism, together with this diagnosis becoming more often than not the responsibility of busy community paediatricians, means 'other approaches' are thin on the ground. They further recommend that: '... diagnosis should distinguish between aggression and other seriously challenging behaviours (which may justify an antipsychotic agent) and lesser levels of irritability (which may not)' (Morgan & Taylor, 2007: 1069). However, they don't explain how a clinician is supposed to differentiate between what one should consider 'seriously' challenging behaviour and 'irritability'. Of most concern, however, is that the evidence they cite to support their position is at best questionable, at worst should lead to the opposite conclusion than that which the authors reach.

In support of their recommendation to use anti-psychotics for challenging behaviour they refer to two studies only (McCracken et al., 2002; Shea et al., 2004). A critical review of these two studies reveals anything but encouraging news for this practice. First, both studies were of only eight weeks in duration, far from the many years for which drugs prescribed to pacify behaviour are usually used. Second, one of the studies (McCracken et al., 2002) reviewed their subjects at six months and found a familiar pattern seen with drug treatment for behavioural problems – that of diminishing returns, with less than half of the group that had received the anti-psychotic now rated as 'improved' (interestingly they do not provide the data for how the placebo group were doing after six months). Third, a decrease in challenging behaviour in those receiving an anti-psychotic at a sufficient dose is really a foregone conclusion, after all anti-psychotics are also classified (more accurately) as 'major tranquillisers'. Whether the effect of 'tranquillisation' is viewed as a therapeutic effect or side effect

depends on your perspective. Reflecting this fact, both studies rated high levels of somnolence (sleepiness or drowsiness), for example, Shea et al. (2004) recorded a 72 per cent rate of somnolence in the group receiving the anti-psychotic and a two-thirds response rate (in terms of a decrease of aggressive behaviours) to the anti-psychotic, leading to the rather peculiar scenario where, arguably, the same pharmacological effect is simultaneously rated as therapeutic (decrease in aggressive behaviours) and an adverse effect (somnolence) – after all you can't get up to much mischief if you're drowsy.

What is most worrying, however, is that the editorial pays little attention to the serious adverse effects of the anti-psychotics, which were prevalent in both studies. To give just one example, both studies found the group receiving the anti-psychotic put on more weight than the group with the placebo; in McCracken et al. (2002), this was an average of 2.7 vs 0.8 Kg, and in the Shea et al. (2004) study this was an average of 2.7 vs 1.0 Kg. Remember, this was after only eight weeks of 'treatment'. Thus these children were being put at a greatly increased risk of serious illnesses such as cardiovascular disease and diabetes.

The second publication (or rather series of publications) is to do with the 'Treatment of Early-Onset Schizophrenia Spectrum Disorders' (TEOSS) study (Sikich et al., 2008). This is a large multi-centre study of anti-psychotics in people aged 8–19 years, with diagnoses of schizophrenia or schizoaffective disorder and funded by the National Institute of Mental Health in the US (though most of the authors disclosed a long list of 'conflicts of interest' including sponsorship by, and speaking for, pharmaceutical companies). This study set out to evaluate the safety and efficacy of three anti-psychotics in comparison with each other (risperidone, olanzapine and molindone) for the treatment of children and adolescents with schizophrenia or schizoaffective disorder (i.e., those considered to be suffering with the most serious psychiatric disorders in the form of a psychosis).

The TEOSS study showed that, even under trial conditions, around half discontinued treatment within eight weeks. The eight-week findings revealed that the likely reasons for such a high drop-out rate so early in the study were poor efficacy and/or high levels of adverse effects. Clinical response was defined as a combination of clinician-identified improvement and a decrease of 20 per cent on a symptom

scale. Clinical response rates were low (below 50 per cent) in all three groups. A significant increase in weight and body mass index led to early discontinuation of the olanzapine treatment arm, with youths taking olanzapine gaining an average of 6.1 kg. The olanzapine group also had significant abnormalities in the heart electrical activity (measured by ECG) and increases in cholesterol, low-density lipoprotein, insulin and liver enzymes. Weight gain was less but still notable (with a mean of about 3.6 kg) in the risperidone group. Molindone was not associated with weight change. Other common adverse events included akathisia (a sense of inner restlessness) in the molindone group and constipation in the risperidone group. Prolactin levels were also increased in the risperidone group (which can lead to breast tissue growth and milk secretion) (Sikich et al., 2008). The remaining two arms of the study (risperidone and molindone) continued for another year. By 12 months, only about 10 per cent of the original study volunteers remained (Findling et al., 2010), a shockingly high attrition rate, making further comparisons and conclusions meaningless given that 90 per cent had effectively 'voted with their feet' and left the study.

So, there is little evidence to support the efficacy of using a medication-centred or medical model-centred approach to helping even those with the more severe forms of disturbances that lead to hearing voices and much evidence to show that they are exposed to a high level of risk. As I have mentioned, part of the widespread justification for the use of psychiatric drugs is the idea that they work by correcting, or helping to correct, underlying biological abnormalities that produce particular psychiatric symptoms (the disease model). This is understandable. Most drugs used in medicine can be understood as working according to a *disease-centred model* – even analgesics, for example, work by acting on the physiological mechanisms that produce pain. In psychiatry, the disease-centred model is reflected in the names of the major drug classes: antidepressants are believed to reverse biochemical pathways that give rise to symptoms of depression and anti-psychotics are thought to act on mechanisms that produce psychotic symptoms. From this viewpoint, the therapeutic actions of drugs (their actions on disease processes) can be distinguished from other effects, accordingly termed side-effects.

An alternative way of understanding (and one supported by more evidence than the disease model as a way of understanding effects of psychiatric drugs on a person's mental health) is a *drug-centred model* of drug action. This stresses that psychiatric drugs are, first and foremost, psychoactive drugs. They induce complex, varied, often unpredictable physical and mental states that patients typically experience as global, rather than distinct therapeutic effects and side-effects. Drugs may be useful because some altered states can suppress the distressing experiences associated with certain mental states such as the effects of 'tranquillisation' in helping manage fear, distress and anger produced by hearing 'persecutory' voices (Moncreiff, 2008b).

Incorporating this second perspective (the drug-centred model) into prescribing medication, means different types of conversation and partnerships can happen between the treating doctor and the young person and their family. We can be more honest about the lack of therapeutic specificity and the risks in terms of side effects. Medication can then be framed, not as a curative or necessary element of the intervention (like insulin would have to be for type-1 diabetes), but as something that may be useful to help manage particular emotional states, particularly those involving unbearably high levels of arousal. My experience in using such an approach is that when I see a young person experiencing voices, more often than not medication is not needed and when we do decide together to use it, it is usually in a pragmatic manner to address a particular problem (such as a sleeping tablet for a few nights to tackle not sleeping for several nights, or a 'major tranquilliser' for a while to help manage distressing and persecutory voices) at a relatively low dose and set up as a time-limited intervention while we work on other things.

CONCLUSION: MEANING AND THERAPEUTIC RELATIONSHIPS

There is a large literature on psychotherapy confirming that it is generally a safe and effective intervention (Wampold, 2001). Recent meta-analyses of decades of outcome studies have concluded that, as regards the 'within treatment' variables, it is the quality of the therapeutic alliance that accounts for most of the within-therapy

variance in treatment outcome and is up to seven times more influential in promoting change than the treatment model used (Duncan et al., 2004). Thus there is a strong empirical case that the non-specific aspects of psychotherapy, or 'know-how' in building a strong therapeutic alliance (which involves being able to engage meaningfully with the young person and their family's beliefs and practices), are more important than specific techniques being used. Bruce Wampold concludes from his meticulous review of the literature that, 'Decades of psychotherapy research have failed to find a scintilla of evidence that any specific ingredient is necessary for therapeutic change' (Wampold, 2001: 204). This provides a strong empirical case for putting the patient's rather than the therapist's technical model in the 'driver's seat' of therapy.

Thus when it comes to giving advice it is not possible to provide a 'cookbook' set of things that a doctor, therapist, young person or their family *should* do. Non-specific factors are important because they represent a wide variety of elements that draw heavily on cultural referents that are shared between clinician and patient. Historically these play a central role within the therapeutic encounter. They invoke hope, trust and faith, themes that consistently emerge as important from service user and carer research and narratives about recovery (see Bracken & Thomas, 2005). There are powerful historical and cultural claims on doctors like myself that make it impossible to disavow the importance of these factors in clinical work. It highlights the need for psychiatrists like myself to attend to the value and significance of culture and meaning and building strong therapeutic alliances that are respectful of the service user's experience and beliefs. Unfortunately, it may, therefore, be easier to conclude with some 'don'ts' rather than 'dos' as the specific therapeutic tasks must emerge in the context of developing a meaningful relationship with the young person and their family. However, in doing so, the research is pointing us toward avoiding the medical model as the primary explanatory model and avoiding medication as the primary form of treatment.

REFERENCES

Angermeyer, MC & Matschinger, H (2005) Causal beliefs and attitudes to people with schizophrenia. Trend analysis based on data from two population surveys in Germany. *British Journal of Psychiatry, 186*, 331–4.

Bracken, P & Thomas, P (2005) *Postpsychiatry: Mental health in a postmodern world.* Oxford: Oxford University Press.

Coleman, R (1999) *Recovery: An alien concept?* Colchester: Handsell.

Crumlish, N, Whitty, P & Kamali, M (2005) Early insight predicts depression and attempted suicide after 4 years in first-episode schizophrenia and schizophreniform disorder. *Acta Psychiatrica Scandinavica, 112*, 449–55.

Duncan, B, Miller, S & Sparks, J (2004) *The Heroic Client.* San Francisco: Jossey-Bass.

Escher, S, Romme, M, Buiks, A, Delespaul, P & van Os, J (2002) Independent course of childhood auditory hallucinations: A sequential 3-year follow-up study. *British Journal of Psychiatry, 181* (suppl. 43), s10–s18.

Findling, RL, Johnson, JL, McClellan, J et al. (2010) Double-blind maintenance safety and effectiveness findings from the treatment of early-onset schizophrenia spectrum (TEOSS) study. *Journal of the American Academy of Child and Adolescent Psychiatry, 49*, 583–94.

Hasson-Ohayon, H, Kravetz, S, Roe, D & David, AS (2006) Insight into psychosis and quality of life. *Comparative Psychiatry, 47*, 265–9.

Hopper, K, Harrison, G, Janka, A & Sartorius, N (eds) (2007) *Recovery from Schizophrenia: An international perspective.* Oxford: Oxford University Press.

McCracken, JT, McGough, J, Shah, B, Cronin, P & Hong, D (2002) Resperidone in children with autism and serious behavioral problems. *New England Journal of Medicine, 347*, 314–21.

McGee, R, Williams, S & Poulton, R (2000) Hallucinations in non-psychotic children. *Journal of the American Academy of Child and Adolescent Psychiatry, 39*, 12–13.

Moncrieff, J (2008a) Neoliberalism and biopsychiatry: A marriage of convenience. In: CI Cohen & S Timimi (eds) *Liberatory Psychiatry: Philosophy, politics, and mental health.* Cambridge: Cambridge University Press.

Moncrieff, J (2008b) *The Myth of the Chemical Cure.* Basingstoke: Palgrave MacMillan.

Morgan, S & Taylor, E (2007) Antipsychotic drugs in children with autism. *British Medical Journal, 334*, 1069–70.

Moynihan, R, Heath, I & Henry, D (2002) Selling sickness: The pharmaceutical industry and disease mongering. *BMJ, 324*, 886–91.

Poulton, R, Caspi, A, Moffitt, TE et al. (2000) Children's self-reported psychotic symptoms and adult schizophreniform disorder: A 15-year longitudinal study. *Archives of General Psychiatry, 57*, 1053–8.

Read, J, Bentall, R & Mosher, L (2004) *Models of Madness: Psychological, social and biological approaches to schizophrenia.* Hove: Routledge.

Read, J, Haslam, N, Sayce, I & Davies, E (2006) Prejudice and schizophrenia: A

review of the 'Mental illness is an illness like any other' approach. *Acta Psychiatrica Scandinavica, 114,* 303–18.

Romme, M (ed) (1996) *Understanding Voices. Coping with auditory hallucinations and confusing realities.* Colchester: Handsell Publications.

Romme, MAJ & Escher, ADMAC (1989) Hearing Voices. *Schizophrenia Bulletin, 15* (2), 209–16.

Romme, M, Escher, S, Dillon, J, Corstens, D & Morris, M (2009) *Living with Voices: 50 stories of recovery.* Ross-on-Wye: (in association with Birmingham City University) PCCS Books.

Shea, S, Turgay, A, Carroll, A, Schulz, M & Orlik, M (2004) Risperidone in the treatment of disruptive behavioral symptoms in children with autistic and other pervasive developmental disorders. *Pediatrics, 114*, e634–41.

Sikich, L, Frazier, JA, McClellan, J et al. (2008) Double-blind comparison of first- and second-generation antipsychotics in early-onset schizophrenia and schizoaffective disorder: Findings from the Treatment of Early-Onset Schizophrenia Spectrum Disorders (TEOSS) study. *American Journal of Psychiatry, 165*, 1420–31.

Thomas, P (1997) *The Dialectics of Schizophrenia.* London: Free Association.

Timimi, S (2008) Child psychiatry and its relationship to the pharmaceutical industry: Theoretical and practical issues. *Advances in Psychiatric Treatment, 14*, 3–9.

Wampold, BE (2001) *The Great Psychotherapy Debate: Models, methods, and findings.* Hillsdale, NJ: Lawrence Erlbaum.

Warner, R (2010) Does the scientific evidence support the recovery model? *The Psychiatrist, 34*, 3–5.

Watters, E (2009) *Crazy Like Us: The globalization of the American psych.* New York: Free Press.

Whitaker, R (2002) *Mad in America.* Cambridge MA: Perseus.

Sami Timimi is a Consultant Child and Adolescent Psychiatrist and Director of Postgraduate Education in the National Health Service in Lincolnshire and a Visiting Professor of Child and Adolescent Psychiatry at the University of Lincoln, UK. He writes from a critical psychiatry perspective on topics relating to mental health and has published many articles in leading journals and chapters in books on many subjects including eating disorders, psychotherapy, behavioural disorders and cross-cultural psychiatry. He has authored four books, *Pathological Child Psychiatry* and the *Medicalization of Childhood*, published in 2002, *Naughty Boys: Anti-Social Behaviour, ADHD and the Role of Culture,* published in 2005, *Misunderstanding ADHD: A Complete Guide for Parents to Alternatives to Drugs,* published in 2007, and *A Straight Talking Introduction to Children's Mental Health Problems* published in 2009. He co-edited with Begum Maitra *Critical Voices in Child and Adolescent Mental Health,* published in 2006, *Liberatory Psychiatry: Philosophy, Politics, and Mental Health,* with Carl Cohen, published in 2008 and *Rethinking ADHD: From Brain to Culture,* with Jonathan Leo in 2009. He has co-authored with Brian McCabe and Neil Gardner *The Myth of Autism: Medicalising Men and Boys' Social and Emotional Competence,* to be published in 2010.

5

The *Maastricht Interview** for Children and Adolescents Hearing Voices: Research results

Hearing voices is a very intrusive experience that can have a strong influence on daily life. To begin with, the presence of the voices is often a confusing and distressing experience; for example, it is difficult to hold a conversation with people when other voices are talking to you at the same time. Dealing with the content of what the voices are saying presents a further difficulty. How do you evaluate this confusion? In 1989, based on the experience of adults who heard voices, we developed a structured interview, with 11 topics, as a format for a dialogue about the experience of voice hearing. We used this interview both in our research and in therapeutic contacts. With the aid of a child psychoanalyst, Mrs. Gijssen-Pinckards, we adapted it for children and adolescents and used this interview in our three-year follow-up study on 80 children between the age of 8–19 years who were hearing voices. We interviewed the children four times, with a year in between each interview. In this article we will discuss the topics of the interview in detail, and use examples to allow some research findings to speak for themselves. Nearly all the interviews were conducted in the presence of at least one or both parents. Research proposal and conclusions are published in separate articles.

It was a patient who first challenged professionals to revise their attitude in relation to auditory hallucinations. The patient, Patsy Hage, heard voices that dominated her and made her feel powerless, she eventually became suicidal. It took her a year to convince her psychiatrist, Marius Romme, that the voices were real to her. The traditional opinion in psychiatry at that time was that to acknowledge people's voices would be colluding with their delusions and it would confuse them more.

* This can be found in full at www.hearing-voices.com

Marius Romme listened to Patsy and decided to test out her insistence that the voices were real to her. He arranged for Patsy to talk about her voices with other people who also heard voices. Comparing their experiences went well, but it soon became obvious that the other voice hearers, who were also patients, felt as powerless as Patsy.

The conclusion was that someone who could cope with hearing voices must be found. Romme and Patsy participated in a very popular television programme and asked people who heard voices to contact them. Of the 500 responses that followed, there were 173 people who could cope with hearing voices, functioned well in daily life and had never been psychiatric patients. In order to get more detailed information, a questionnaire was designed and a pilot study conducted. The three most important findings of the study were that some people who heard voices were able to cope with them; the onset of the voices is often related to a traumatic event or a situation in which a person is powerless and, thirdly; the voices are personal and they have a personal message.

These elements form four of the topics that are part of the *Maastricht Interview*: the acceptance of the voices; to learn to talk about them; to learn to cope with them; to learn to understand their message. All these elements should be focused on in the therapeutic process.

DIALOGUE

The *Maastricht Interview* is a tool that opens a dialogue and is a means of encouraging talking about the voice-hearing experience in which both the voice hearer and the interviewer gain knowledge. It is an open dialogue, during which experiences will be discussed and no conclusions will be made. Voice hearers often find that as soon as they start to talk about their voices, people around them do not know how to react. In a therapeutic setting, the value of the experience of the voice hearer is often not acknowledged or is viewed very negatively. This is understandable because therapists' ideas are based on the patients they meet. These are mainly voice hearers who cannot cope with their experience and are looking for psychiatric help. However, it is only a

certain group of people who look for psychiatric help; therapists mostly never meet the non-patients, people who cope with hearing voices as part of their normal daily life.

Several studies on student populations and epidemiological studies found prevalence of voice hearing in the general population of about two per cent. With children and adolescents, an even higher rating of about eight per cent was found (Sidgewick, 1894; West, 1948; Green et al., 1973; Posey & Losch, 1983; Bentall & Slade, 1985; Young et al., 1986; Romme & Escher, 1989; Tien, 1991; Barrett & Etheridge, 1992; McGee et al., 2000, Bijl et al., 1998). One might conclude that it is not the presence of the voices that is pathological, but the way in which people cope with them.

The lack of knowledge about the non-patient group is a consequence of the taboo surrounding hearing voices that prevents most people from talking freely about them. People who can cope with their voices prefer not to talk about them because, within our Western culture, hearing voices is still frequently seen as a symptom of a mental illness.

The taboo and the association with an illness prevent people from learning about their experience. In order to start coping, one must be able to talk about voice hearing: to explore the experience, to look for a structure, to look for the message of the voices and to look for triggers that may induce the voices. The *Maastricht Interview* attempts to make the experience into a personal study that allows this process. It can unfold a story that is understandable to both the voice hearer and other people.

The questions structure the experience and can give rise to new questions about which the voice hearer has never previously thought; for example, triggers and coping mechanisms. For therapists, the interviewer can give information about: the possible relationship with the voices and the life history of the voice hearer, about underlying problems, the influence of the voices in daily life and the power structure between the voice hearer and the voice(s).

In this article, quantitative and qualitative data will be used from the children's research to illustrate the kind of information that the 11 interview topics might give. The word 'children' will be used, meaning the whole population of children between 8 and 19 years of age.

NATURE OF THE EXPERIENCE

Questions on the first topic are about the nature of the experience. Is the experience to be categorised as an auditory hallucination and, apart from hearing voices, are other unusual experiences present? Under this heading the children were asked:

- Do you hear the voices in the head or through the ears?
- Do you think that the voices are 'not-me' (ego-dystonic)?
- Are the voices sleep related (heard when falling asleep or waking up)?
- Do you have other experiences like visions, auras, sounds or music?
- Are you able to hold a dialogue with the voices?

All children participating in our research heard voices that were ego-dystonic. Most of them had an argument such as, 'It must be someone else, because I do not say such stupid things' or 'I hear two voices, I cannot be two voices myself'. Most of the children believed that others could not hear their voices. Often they had checked it with the people around them. Only one child thought that another person might hear his voices, however he could not identify that person and has never met him.

Nature of the experience	
Hear voices in the head only	67%
Hear voices through the ears	33%
Hear voices during daytime as well as sleep-related voices	27%
Hear voices during daytime only	73%
Other experiences:	
Have visions	65%

VISIONS

In this research, the emphasis is on hearing voices. We do not have quantitative figures about the interpretation of the visions, but there is an impression based on the interviews; 65 per cent of the children saw visions. These varied from vague shadows to very clear images. Not all visions were described as frightening. During the interviews it became apparent that, in most cases, it was the individual interpretation of the vision that produced fear and anxiety or otherwise in the children. Some children reported seeing coloured auras. They were initially afraid of these because they did not know what these colours meant.

A good example of the relationship between visions and anxiety is that of a child that said that she was not afraid of the vision of deer ripped apart and bleeding. This vision would frighten anyone. Visions are not always associated with a voice or a sound: 39 per cent of the children reported seeing a vision and hearing a voice or sound at the same time. About 50 per cent of the children heard voices as well as sounds like the slamming of a door, or a garden gate or hearing music.

CHARACTERISTICS OF THE VOICES

In this topic, extensive questions were asked about the characteristics of the five most important voices. The children were asked:

- the number of voices and the name of the five most important voices
- the gender, age
- tone of the voice
- frequency of the voice
- whether the voices resemble someone known to the hearer

These questions are asked because in our research on adults we found that:

- voices with a clear identity might give an indication of past trauma

or a situation that makes the voice hearer powerless

- characteristics of the voices, like gender and age, might give an indication the identity of the person involved in the trauma
- voices might be positive and offer advice
- a clear identity of the voice might offer more possibilities to develop a different (the voice hearer's own) opinion

For therapists, the characteristics might give an indication of the kind of trauma and the people involved. For example, a male child reported that he heard the voice of his teacher. His problem appeared to be this teacher. The boy's father was a soldier who had been sent to Bosnia. The boy could not cope with this. After his father was sent abroad, the child never talked about him. However, on one occasion at school, when he did try to speak about his father, the teacher ridiculed him about it. A short while later, the boy started to hear the voice of the teacher who had ridiculed him.

In another case, it emerged that one girl who had been sexually abused by the boy next door and two of his friends, started to hear voices that had the same tone of voice and were the same age and gender as the boys who had abused her.

The experience of using the interview showed that one should not make assumptions or jump to conclusions on the first information. It is better to finish the whole interview before attempting an analysis.

For example, an 11-year-old boy heard a female and a male voice, who quarrelled about him. When asked a question at school that he could not answer, the male voice gave him incorrect advice. Then the female voice told the boy this was not the right answer and both voices started to quarrel, which confused the boy. During the interview the boy was asked whether the female voice was always right. He answered: 'Mostly, she is. Not in traffic.' Within five minutes, his mother disclosed that she did not like driving, as she was not very skillful in traffic. On first impressions there seemed to be a connection between the parents and the voices the child heard, suggesting that there could be a problematic situation. However, in the third year of the research it emerged that the child's IQ was 85, much to low for the school he was attending, causing him a lot of stress.

NUMBER OF VOICES

Analysis showed that the number of voices each child heard had no influence on how they coped with the voices or their continuation or discontinuation. We concluded that coping with hearing only one voice was no easier than coping with a number of voices, or that hearing only one voice made it more likely that the voice would disappear. In the first interview, we found that most children heard less than five voices.

One voice	21%
Between two and five voices	37%
Between six and ten voices	17%
More than ten voices	20%
Changing number of voices	5%

The number of voices was asked as well as the characteristics of the five most important voices. For the majority of children it was the same voice. They were mostly male voices; only 40 per cent had a name.

The most important voice was a male voice of someone 30–40 years (about the age of their father)	60–70%
Always the same voice	70%
The voice had a name	40%

Identity of the most important voice, the children reported:

Unknown	65.4%
Father	2.5%
Mother	1.2%
Sister/brother	2.4%
Grandfather	2.5%
Grandmother	2.5%
Deceased person	2.5%
Themselves	4.9%
Teacher	1.2%

Friend	1.2%
Alien/computer	3.7%
Different from above*	9.9%

 *(Robot, ghost, phantom, spook, beast)

Characteristics of the voices

Overall tone of the voices:

Friendly	25%
Aggressive or unpleasant	50%
Neutral (neither positive nor negative)	25%

FREQUENCY

In the analysis, we found that the frequency was very important; a high frequency was a predictor of the continuation of the voices. The more often the voices were heard, the more the likelihood they would not disappear.

Frequency of hearing voices

Daily	60%
Continuous	10%
Every hour	13%
Every week	20%
(varying from once to several times)	
Every month	3%
(varying from once to several times)	
Changing frequency	17%
(voices might be heard sometimes, often, and sometimes rarely)	

TRIGGERS

Time, place and activity related to voice hearing: In the interview, we distinguished two categories of triggers to hearing voices. The first category was related to the time, place and activity when the voices were heard. Generally, it was not difficult for the children to talk about these triggers.

Emotions related to voice hearing: The second category was related to emotions such as aggression, anger, sadness, being tired, anxiety, doubt, jealousy, being happy. Talking about emotional triggers was more difficult. The structure of the interview enabled talking about emotional triggers to build up. In the daily life of the children, we often saw a combination of both categories. For example, some children reported that they were afraid at night in their own bedroom, when it was dark, or they were afraid to walk in the street on their own.

Time, place and activity related voices
When a question on this topic was answered with 'yes', it might indicate that there was a problem in this specific area. In therapy, it is wise to check whether there is a relationship between triggers and possible problems in this area. For example, in our research, we found that quite a lot of children heard voices at school. These children experienced problems at school, which people around them were not always aware of. For example, they were bullied by their peers or dealt with unfairly by their teacher. For example, a teacher had put a girl who had a hearing impairment to the back of the classroom. Not only was she unable to hear what he said, she also had too much time to spend with the voices and started to talk to them out loud.

A number of children were having ability problems. Their inability to cope with some subjects in the school curriculum resulted in some children behaving aggressively. Their feelings of powerlessness and inability to cope at school were continually influenced by the voices. The results of the research showed that, sometimes, changes in the circumstances that triggered the voices might make the voices disappear. For example, a number of children reported that the voices disappeared when they changed schools because of their ability problems or because they went from primary school to secondary school.

Because the children were interviewed four times they became more familiar with the interview topics. In the time between the interviews, parents and children discussed them and some parents came to their own conclusions. For one mother the connection between the problems her daughter experienced at school with her peers and the voices was so clear that she told the interviewer: 'I would not be surprised if the voices are gone next year when she changes school'. She was proved to be right.

More insight into what triggers the voices creates the possibility of organising more efficient support for the children. For example, in the case of the girl who saw visions and heard a voice in her bedroom and became so afraid that she did not want to go to bed, her family took her seriously and her father went to her bedroom every night to look in her closet and under her bed to see whether there was a voice or a vision. As he found none, he told her and she was satisfied and was able to go to bed. However, a problem arose with the early darkness of winter. The girl liked to take long showers and insisted that a family member wait outside the shower room in the corridor, so she could feel safe. No one wanted to do this. Eventually her mother worked out a solution; she would call her for her shower at four o'clock when it was still daylight.

Support such as this is important, as long as it is within reason. When limits are exceeded, other problems can arise, for example, if parents allow their child to sleep in their bed when they are afraid of the voices. One father complained about his ten-year-old daughter, who slept between him and his wife for four years. As her size increased with age, she took up more and more space in the bed. The father eventually had to sleep on the edge of the bed. His daughter often could not bear heat and threw the duvet off the bed. She had become a child that dominated his marriage as well as his sleep and had not learned to cope with her voices independently of her parents.

Emotional triggers

The second category is emotional triggers. In the interview there is a whole list of them, corresponding with the emotions voice hearers mentioned in the pilot study. The list is always carried out systematically. This systematic approach has been found to help reveal unexpected factors that might explain certain behaviours of the children.

Firstly, we asked whether the voices came when the children felt particular emotions. Secondly, we asked what were the effects of emotions on the voice on these occasions? Did the voices intensify the emotion in a positive or negative way? Or did they just come? Therefore, the questions obtain information about the presence of emotions in relation to the appearance of the voices, as well as the reaction of the child on the presence of emotion combined with the voices. Some children said that when they are angry the voices help them by saying: 'Do you think this is wise? Do you have to be so angry?' Most children reported that when they are angry, the voices make them feel angrier. Sometimes voices can cause some children to exceed limits; for example, a very slim good-looking girl who said that she became so angry that she pushed a woman over her shopping trolley.

The emotional triggers often appear to have the same hold as the triggers of time, place and activity. If the voices appear with particular emotions, there might well be problems with these feelings. For example, Ben is 11 years old; he has never been in residential care because of hearing voices. In the first interview, Ben said that he could become so angry that he was afraid that he would start a fight. He thought that he was so strong that he would probably knock the person down. This reasoning put Ben into an impossible position. Instead of becoming angry himself, he made other people angry. At the first interview a very angry mother aided by an uncle was present.

In the third year of the research Ben accidentally found a teacher who could help him. Ben explained that one of his classmates bullied him and this made him become so angry that he did not know what to do about his anger. He was afraid that if he started to fight with the boy he would knock him down. The teacher invited both Ben and the classmate for a talk. In the presence of the teacher, the boys were forced to explain to each other what provoked their disagreements and they had to find a compromise. They had to make a deal and shake hands to show each other that they meant it seriously. This solution worked well; every time Ben felt angry and he felt that he could not cope with it, he consulted the teacher. When he became very angry at home he went voluntarily to his bedroom and stayed there until he calmed down. During the previous year, his parents sent him to his room as a punishment.

In the final interview, Ben reported that he could cope better with aggression by carrying out an internal dialogue. When he became angry he would say to himself: 'Do sit down, it can only get worse.'

Some of the children in the study were unable to learn how to cope with emotion in the way Ben had. However, they learned to cope with the help of professional care. In Holland, the ambulatory care unit and some private therapists provide assertiveness training. Through this training, the children who frequently felt angry learned to express themselves in different ways. Consequently, they did not explode with anger, but could talk about their feelings and express them safely.

It is striking that not only the presence of certain emotions, but their absence, can indicate certain problems. One girl reported that she was never angry. She said: 'Whenever I start feeling angry, the voices come. I never get angry.' In group therapy, she learned to feel anger. She had to explain to other group members certain disturbing experiences, why they had happened and why she could not react. The therapist would repeatedly say 'I have not fully understood what you are explaining'. The child had to tell the story repeatedly until she felt the emotions connected to the incident that she was relating.

Two frequent triggers for voices were doubt and uncertainty. The voices repeatedly interfered with and ridiculed the children's decisions, sometimes with far-reaching consequences. One girl reported that she only bought black clothes. 'The voices want me to buy them. I don't even like black!' she said. Another child, a boy, reported that the voices decided what he should put on his bread. It had begun with him asking for advice from his voices and it ended with their total dominance. The voices only allowed him to eat what they said he should eat. If he did not listen, they would punish him.

However, the opposite also happened. Some children who began to ask their voices for advice found they could rely on it. Whenever they did not know what to choose or, for example, what to wear, they asked the voices. One girl heard her voice say; 'I would rather put those red shoes on, they go nicely with your dress.' She put the dress and shoes together and agreed. Children who cope with the voices in this way are not usually in residential care. They learned to be critical and discerning about what the voices said and decided whether they could use the advice or whether it would give them trouble.

Place, time and activity as triggers

The triggers – place, time and activity – scored less often than the emotional triggers.

The voice appears:	
In a certain place – at home or at school	52%
With certain activities, like doing homework or playing outside	44%
At certain times, like the weekend or going to bed	38%

Although 50 per cent of the children were not in psychiatric care, most children were afraid of the voices. The triggers anxiety, fear and sadness scored highly. Nearly 50 per cent of the children mentioned being alone as a trigger. In the research, 'being alone' is not seen as part of the categories of place, activity or time; it was put under the topic 'emotional trigger'. Some children reported that 'being alone' was positive while others felt it was negative.

Emotional triggers	
Anxiety	70%
Anger	54%
Sadness	50%
Being alone	49%
Doubt	40%
Uncertainty	46%
Feeling unhappy	36%
Feeling guilty	35%
Being tired	29%

HISTORY OF VOICE HEARING

In our research with adults hearing voices (Romme & Escher, 1989), we found that 70 per cent of people started to hear voices in relation to a trauma or to an emotionally overpowering situation. One of the research questions in the children's research was, therefore, whether

this was also the case with children. With adults, we saw that, if they were able to see a relationship between the voices and a possible trauma, this had a positive influence on their way of coping with the voices. By relating the voices to their life history, the experience became more understandable and less alien.

Under the topic 'history of voice hearing' is a checklist with 18 life events that could make a person powerless and could be experienced as traumatic; the death of a grandmother, grandfather or a friend, divorce of parents, moving house, changing schools, etc. In the pilot study, many adults and children reported that events such as these preceded the onset of their voice hearing.

The checklist is systematic and the first question asked is whether the child has experienced a particular event. The second question asked whether the particular event triggered the onset of the voices. In cases where the voice hearing preceded the trauma, we asked whether the event had changed the nature of the voices. Therapists who have used this method with a patient they thought they knew well have been surprised to hear things, many things which they previously did not know.

In the research setting, a girl had begun to hear a voice at the age of six at the time that her grandmother died. The voice was friendly and supportive. When she was 11 years old, the voice changed and she began to hear more voices. Gradually the voices became very negative and destructive. In the first interview, the girl said nothing traumatic had happened to her. However, before the second interview she had an informal discussion with the interviewer during which she tested the interviewer to see if she could trust her by asking her opinion about voice hearing and unusual beliefs. Later, during the formal interview, talking about life events, she reported that, when she was 12, she had had a boyfriend of 23, who gave her drugs and let his friends sexually abuse her. She had never told anyone about this incident because she felt that she was to blame.

A boy, Elliot, started to hear positive voices at a time when several things happened to him. His family moved to a temporary house. The school year ended and he expected to go to the same school as his brother, but was not admitted because of a clerical error made by his teacher. Six months before his first interview, the voices had become

negative. The boy became aggressive and was referred to the school GP. The doctor had heard about our research and advised Elliot to participate in it. In the first interview, Elliot told that us that the voices had suddenly become negative. The interviewer asked Elliot and his mother, who was present, to return in their thoughts to the time this had happened. Suddenly they both knew what had happened.

One Saturday Elliot had accompanied his mother, brother and his brother's friend to a football ground. This friend played in goal and tried to stop a ball, but missed it and fell into a window. The glass cut his arms, the boy suffered arterial bleeding and nearly died. Elliot's brother and mother offered first aid, while Elliot went to the parking lot to clear it for the ambulance. In the following weeks, Elliot's mother and brother talked a lot about the event, never mentioning Elliot's role. Remembering the event caused him and his mother to talk about it in detail. In this discussion, the mother admitted that it was strange that she had never involved him in previous discussions about the event. She realised she had not paid enough attention to what Elliot had done. She shared the new feelings with him and, in the next year, both the voices and his aggressive behaviour disappeared.

Of the 80 children participating in the research, 62 per cent reported that they recognised a relationship between the voices and at least one traumatic event. Some children reported more than one trauma. Statistically we saw that children who had experienced more than one trauma were more likely to look for psychiatric care.

INFLUENCE OF THE VOICES

What influence does hearing voices have in daily life? Do they only have influence at home, only at school, only in social contacts or do they influence all levels of daily life? This topic contains 13 items. From the interviews we know that the voices scare the children, cause them to pick quarrels and fights, to steal, to lie, disturb doing homework, etc. Notwithstanding these negative consequences, the influence of voices can also be positive. The voices can give support, advice and counsel. They might suggest for example, 'Shouldn't you do your homework, because it is nearly bedtime?'

Events precipitating the onset of voices, in four categories

	Total %	N
1. Confrontation with death		
Total	22.5%	18
2. Problems at home		
Serious tension with parents and or brothers/sisters	10%	
Divorced parents	6%	
Moving house	3%	
Total	23.7%	19
3. Problems concerning the school situation		
Capability problems	9%	
Changing schools	7%	
Being bullied	3%	
Total	23.7%	19
4. Other kinds of trauma/problems		
Sexual abuse	4%	
A problem with health and long hospital stays	4%	
Birth trauma	2%	
Seeing something weird	3%	
Rejection in love	1%	
Abortion	1%	
Narcotics	1%	
Brain damage caused by traffic accident	1%	
Total	21.2%	17
No trauma		
Total	13.7%	11

It is striking that about 50 per cent of the children hear positive voices (as well as negative). In questioning the influence of voices, we had discussions with the children about the consequences on their own behaviour. Some children reported that the voices made them so angry that they started to quarrel with their siblings or withdraw to their bedroom.

Two examples show that this line of questioning might be more important for parents in explaining the child's behaviour than for the child itself. During an interview, one child, a girl, ignored the interviewer but said directly to her father: '... that is why I could not play chess with you yesterday. The voices forbade me to.' On another occasion, a boy turned around to his mother and said, '... that is why I always wait to go to the toilet until you go to the kitchen at night. The voice might be in the corridor leading to the toilet.'

During the research period, it became clear that, as the behaviour of the child became more understandable to the parents, they became more tolerant towards the children. The children began to feel less insecure and showed affection more openly. Some parents explained the changes between the child and themselves as: 'My child has become like one of the other children. They are no longer singled out as "the voice-hearing child". I also allow myself to become angry again when something is not right.'

Analyses of the first interviews showed that the voices considerably influenced all the children's daily life. Seventy per cent of the children experienced problems at home because of the voices. Eighty-two per cent experienced problems at school. Most of the children (80 per cent) were afraid of the voices. Problems in the home included extremely aggressive behaviour. One boy threatened his brother with a knife, another boy hit a glass window so hard that it broke and cut his wrist. At school, problems that arose were mainly lack of concentration, not paying attention to the teacher and getting confused by the voices who twisted answers or turned figures round. The voices distracted the children and demanded attention. Some children responded by talking out loud to the voices.

In the second year, 57 children still heard voices, however the influence of the voices had diminished immensely. Fewer children experienced problems thought to be voice related: at home 33 per cent;

at school 42 per cent. In the following table, the data of the 57 children still hearing voices in the second year were compared with the first year.

Influence of the voices		
Influence of the voices	First year	Second year (N = 57)
Frightening	78%	42%
Confusing	66%	54%
Concentration problems	63%	35%
Provoked quarrels	52%	32%
Disturbed while doing homework	38%	19%
Got punished (by following commands of the voices)	42%	21%
Made them do things they did not want to do	54%	46%
Made them run away	15%	7%

INTERPRETATION OF THE VOICES

Our research with adults showed that most people looked for their own explanation or cause for the voices. Their explanation was often different from that of their therapist. Hardly any voice hearer reported that they thought the voices were an illness. We also found that, if a therapist rejected the explanation of the voice hearer, this influenced the therapeutic relationship and it became more of a battlefield between the two parties. With adults, we saw that the personal explanation was important as it helped them to accept the voices and gave the experience a frame of reference, or belief system, to fit into. Having found a belief system, they acquired the language to explain their experience; it became possible to discuss the experience with other people. The more socially acceptable the explanation, the easier it seemed to be to accept the voices. One of the present research questions was whether this was the case with children.

From the interview, we saw that children were not as interested as adults in finding an explanation. Parents appeared to find it more important; to many parents, to explain the voices as a 'gift' was more acceptable than to call it an illness. Most parents explained the voices as 'paranormal' or a 'special gift'. Some mothers even started training in the paranormal field in order to understand their child better.

Questions in this topic are important for the organisation of support; for example, in the first interview Eric reacted physically when he talked about the voices. He started to sweat and looked very pale. He could hardly talk about his experiences and struggled to find words to describe them. During the interview, his mother said she believed that he was specially gifted. On hearing this, the father, who had just entered the room said, 'Nonsense! He is just a nerd. He can hardly ride his bicycle.' Fortunately for Eric, his mother did not accept his father's explanation. In the second year, his mother thought that he needed care and consulted the family GP, who did not know a lot about hearing voices (which is normal for many GPs) and wanted to refer Eric to a psychiatrist. The mother did not agree to this and found a paranormal therapist who practised group therapy with children who hear voices. In the second year, Eric showed no physical reactions and was able to talk clearly about his experiences. Throughout the research, Eric and his mother visited the therapist regularly, even though they have to travel for hours to see her.

Although most of the children explained the voices as a paranormal gift, there were quite a number that related the voices to the 'other world' or ghosts. Only three per cent of the children thought it was an illness; all of these children were in psychiatric care.

Explanation of the voices	
It is a paranormal gift	39%
A ghost	20%
They come from the other world	18%
Religion	16%
An illness (all these children are in care)	3%
Other explanations (like a doll, robot, etc.)	20%

RELATIONSHIPS WITH THE VOICES

The questions under this topic are meant to make the child aware that he/she has a relationship with the voices. Having a relationship means that there are two parties involved who influence each other. As in every relationship, it is a question of action and reaction. In this case, for example, if the voice hearer allows the voices to exceed small limits, the voices will expand their territory. If the voice hearer lets them know that she/he is not impressed by their punishment, the voices seem to know they do not have enough power. Because of the, often, negative content of the messages of the voices, voice hearers do not like to think in terms of a relationship. They have not chosen this relationship; the voices have been imposed on them. However, to use an analogy, you may have unpleasant neighbours, but you also have to have a relationship with them, whatever form it may take, from ignoring them to trying to get along with them. It is more a question of acknowledging the situation and trying to have as much as influence as possible to improve the situation.

In our research with adults, we found that voice hearers who had never been in psychiatric care described the voices as positive or as mostly positive. They had a relationship in which they felt as powerful as the voices. In most cases, they were able to summon the voices as well as to send them away. If the voices gave them information they did not like, they sent the voices away, ignored the information or thought about it and only used it if it seemed relevant. In their relationship with the voices, they kept their own identity.

With the psychiatric patient groups, this was not the case. They perceived the voices as mostly negative. They were often so afraid of the voices that they did not dare to be critical of the content and did whatever the voices asked them to do. People who were made powerless by the voices often did not realise that they had a relationship in which their own actions and reactions also determined the relationship.

The questions under this topic supply information about how active or passive the voices hearer is in their relationship with the voices. A relationship is subjective and will change as soon as the balance of power changes. During the children's research, we often

saw it happen. In this topic, to determine the level of the power relationship we asked whether the voices listen to the child, agree with him/her, if the child is able to refuse a command of the voices, if they are able to call the voices or if the voices can make them so afraid that they feel totally powerless.

Power relation with the voices	
Voice listens	48%
Child is able to refuse commands	37%
Child is able to call the voice	30%
Child is paralysed by fear of the voices	19%
Child is more powerful than the voices	42%

Children who were able to summon the voices and could refuse their commands were less handicapped by the voices. The children who heard negative voices and who listened to them, were less bothered by the voices than were the children who felt overpowered by the voices. From the literature (Chadwick & Birchwood, 1994; Watkins, 2008) and from our own research (Escher et al., 2002) we saw that the power that the voice hearer attributes to the voices has an influence on the continuation or discontinuation of the voices.

We compared the children's opinion about the voices that they heard in the second year with their opinion of the voices that they heard in the first year.

Attribution of the voices		
Voices are experienced as:	First year	Second year (N = 57)
Predominantly negative	63%	59%
Predominantly positive	17%	24%
Changing	20%	7%

In the analysis, we see that about 50 per cent of the children hear positive voices. There is no significant difference between the patient and the non-patient groups. This confirms the finding that it is largely

the attributes the voice hearer gives to the voices that dominate his/her behaviour towards the voices. For example, a child heard voices that commanded him to destroy the things he liked. Although he perceived the voice as negative, he was not afraid of the voice. Overall, he does not think the voices are negative.

COPING

Questions under this topic are meant to obtain more information about the way that the children cope with the voices. It is not only about how active or passive the voice hearer is, but also about how many coping strategies the child uses. Voice hearers who are made powerless by the voices often used one ineffective form of coping.

This topic can help the children to think about the way they cope. Are the strategies they use effective or ineffective? There are many coping strategies; maybe they would like to try another one?

We distinguished three categories:

- cognitive strategies, such as sending the voices away or making a deal with the voices, listening selectively, thinking about something else and scolding the voices;
- behavioural strategies, such as doing something, closing yourself off from the voices, distraction, or keeping a diary;
- physiological strategies like medication, eating sweets or food.

Differentiation between active and passive coping is made. Active coping is sending the voices away, listening selectively and making a deal with the voices, seeking distraction, keeping a diary. Passive coping is ignoring the voices, scolding them and carrying out rituals.

Some children became very creative and found their own ways of coping. For instance, one boy adapted a computer game. In a labyrinth, a round eating ball would chase an object. He imagined this object was his voice. As he played the game, the round ball ate his voice. Another boy heard two robots. He made a drawing of the robots and a big hypodermic syringe. In his fantasy he gave the metal men an injection and they disappeared. One girl was afraid of a vision of a huge black

bear. Her mother, a voice hearer herself, advised the girl to wash the bear until he was white. The child did as her mother suggested and it helped, as she was not afraid of a white bear.

This topic should stimulate and encourage the children and the therapist to become creative; to look at which strategies work and which do not. The first interview showed that the 80 children participating in the research used a total of 193 coping strategies between them, showing that most children used more than one.

Most-used coping strategies	
	$N = 193$
Distraction	33
Sending the voices away	28
Ignoring the voices	28
Listening to the voices	25
Started doing something (reading, watching television)	23
Going to someone	20
Scolding the voices	19
Thinking about something else	17

HISTORY OF CARE

In this topic, the history of care in relation to the voices is inventoried. We asked what forms of care the children received; from which therapist and from which profession and whether the children were satisfied with the care they received. The data was quite revealing; this topic elicited too much data for discussion in this article.

Statistically we found that whether the children were receiving psychiatric care or not had no influence on the continuation or discontinuation of the voices. On a qualitative level, we found there were differences in the responses of the children, depending on the relationship between the child and the therapist. It appeared that the relationship with the therapist was more important than the technique the therapist used.

SOCIAL NETWORK

The data from the adult research showed that voice hearers who had never been in care received more support at home. Moreover, people around them were aware that they heard voices; it was no secret and these people could talk openly about their experience with other people. Therefore, we wanted to know if the same happened to the children.

   In this topic we made an inventory of the ten most important people, in the opinion of the voice hearer, who know about the voices and with whom they dared to talk about the voices. Sometimes there was surprising information. For instance, some children who did not find one or more siblings or a father important, had to be left out. A detail: 28 per cent of the children had one or more family members who heard voices as well.

   Being able to talk about the voices is important in intimate relations. Some children reported that they did not dare to tell their girlfriend or boyfriend about the voices. These relationships mostly did not last.

REFERENCES

Barrett, TR & Etheridge, JB (1992) Verbal hallucinations in normal 1: People who hear 'voices'. *Applied Cognitive Psychology, 6,* 379–87.

Bentall, RP & Slade, PD (1985) Reality testing in auditory hallucinations: A signal detection analysis. *British Journal of Clinical Psychology, 24,* 159–69.

Bijl, RV, Ravelli, A & Van Zessen, G (1998) Prevalence of psychotic disorder in the general population: Results from The Netherlands mental health survey and incidence study. *Social Psychiatry Epidemology, 33,* 587–96.

Chadwick, P & Birchwood, M (1994) The omnipotence of voices: A cognitive approach to auditory hallucinations. *British Journal of Psychiatry, 164,* 190–201.

Escher, A, Romme, M, Buiks, A, Delespaul, P & van Os, J (2002) Independent course of childhood auditory hallucinations: A sequential 3-year follow-up study. *British Journal of Psychiatry, 181* (suppl. 43), s10–18.

Green, EL et al. (1973) Some methods of evaluating behavioural variations in children 6 to 18. *Journal of the American Academy of Child Psychiatry, 12* (3), 531–53.

McGee, R, Williams, S & Poulton, R (2000) Hallucinations in nonpsychotic children (letter, comments). *Journal of American Academic Child and Adolescent Psychiatry, 39* (1), 12–13.

Posey, TB & Losch, ME (1983) Auditory hallucinations of hearing voices in 375 normal subjects. *Imagination, Cognition and Personality, 3* (2), 99–113.

Romme, MAJ & Escher, ADMAC (1989) Hearing voices. *Schizophrenia Bulletin, 15,* (2), 209–16.

Romme, MAJ, & Escher, ADMAC (eds) (1993) *Accepting Voices.* London: Mind

Romme, MAJ & Escher, ADMAC (2000) *Making Sense of Voices.* London: Mind.

Romme, MAJ, Honig, A, Noorthoorn, O & Escher, ADMAC (1992) Coping with voices: An emancipatory approach. *British Journal of Psychiatry, 161,* 99–103.

Sidgewick, HA et al. (1894) Report of the census of hallucinations. *Proceedings of the Society of Psychiatric Research, 26,* 259–394.

Tien, AY (1991) Distributions of hallucination in the population. *Social Psychiatry and Psychiatric Epidemiology, 26,* 287–92.

Watkins, J (2008) *Hearing Voices: A common human experience.* Melbourne: Hill of Content.

Young, HF, Bentall, RP, Slade, PD & Dewey, ME (1986) Disposition towards hallucination, gender and EPQ score. A brief report. *Personality and Individual Differences, 7* (2), 247–9.

6

Exploring the Experience with the *Maastricht Interview*

In our study the interview was fundamental. It is a systematic way of mapping the experience of children. Mapping the experience helps to make sense of it: what the triggers are and if there is a relationship with problems. Through the years we noticed that a systematic approach is the best way to learn all the facts about the voices which will help in coping with them and with the emotions relating to them.

However, interviewing is not always easy, particularly when you are scared of the voices and/or you have a close relationship with the child. That should not be a reason for not trying. The interview itself has been added to our website. In order to help we added 'The art of interviewing'. This advice is as much for parents as for professionals.

THE ART OF INTERVIEWING

If asked, everybody thinks that he/she can do an interview. In practice, we discovered, through the stories of voice hearers, that this is not the case. The ground for the interview is set before it begins. The voice hearer must feel that he/she can trust the interviewer; that the interviewer will have an ear that listens and a mind that doesn't judge. Talking about the voices is talking about emotions; the interviewee's voices might react to this. However, it is quite normal and should not be seen as exceptional and therefore become frightening. This information should be given after the interview: we always give a telephone number where the voice hearer can reach us in the first 24 hours in case he/she has become disturbed by the interview and wants to discuss anything about it. Hearing voices is

often a confusing experience for which voice hearers have no language. Sometimes a voice hearer, who has never had much opportunity to talk about their voices, opens up too much. He/she might give so much information that it is confusing for the interviewer. From experience, we know that if the interviewer states before the interview that the interviewee will be interrupted whenever the answers are too far away from the line of questioning, that this does not interfere with the interview.

It is important to understand that, during the interview, the interviewer should not make interpretations as this might disturb the process. The purpose of the interview is to collect information about the experience and to hold a dialogue in which the experience and opinion of the voice hearer is central. Interpretation might scare the voice hearer. Many voice hearers know from past experience that, as soon as they talk about their voices, people react in a very negative way. They might not believe the voice hearer, or might see him/her as mentally ill. For a valuable interview, you need the trust of the voice hearer; without trust, they will withhold information and that is not helpful for recovery.

The length of the interview depends on the skill of the interviewer. A skilled interviewer will take about 90 minutes. One might want to conduct the interview in more than one session. For the process of relating the experience to the life history it is important to have all the information, to conduct the whole interview before one makes conclusions. It may sound simple, but for people with training in a therapeutic educational background, it seems to be very difficult not to interpret information and make it into a diagnosis or recommend therapy, for example, in the case of a bereavement.

One more piece of advice: when interviewing a voice hearer, be clear about your own ideas, emotions and fears on the subject. They are part of your personality which you cannot hide.

What we do with the interview

For parents, it is enough just to conduct the interview. Professionals can deal with the information that is given. We developed a format that allows room for further therapy schedules.

From interview to report to construct (Romme & Escher, 2000)
(This section is mainly for professionals.) The first thing to do is to make a report containing all the information from the interview (Romme & Escher, 2000). The report is a summary of about 500 words in which all the topics are mentioned and together they are enough to make sense of the voices in the voice hearer's life. It should give enough information to make the influence of the voices in the interviewee's life understandable: the triggers to the voices and the relationship with trauma or underlying problems. By building a rapport with the interviewee one can learn how much, and which information, is important. In the beginning, people tend to make the report too short or too long.

The report is talked through with the voice hearer; they begin to understand and accept their experience. We found that using quotes from the voice hearer helped to make a report that is accepted by the voice hearer as his or her story. When the voice hearer agrees with the report, the therapist will use it as a construct and an intervention schedule. The construct is a kind of social diagnosis. Hopefully, it makes the relationship between the voices and the life history understandable to the voice hearer.

Information that is used is:

1. the identity of the voices
2. the characteristics of the voices
3. the triggers
4. the onset of the voices (or the change from positive to negative voices)
5. the young person's history

Within the construct two questions are important. Firstly, who do the voices represent? Secondly, what problems do they indicate? The identity and characteristics of the voices will answer the first question. The onset of the voices and the history of the child will answer the second question.

The report, construct and intervention schedule and therapy phases are too complicated to explain in detail here. The book *Making Sense of Voices*, published by Mind, gives very detailed information

(Romme & Escher, 2000). Although the book is based on the adult study, the interview, report and construct hold true for children, as do the interventions, which will help to change the relationship with the voices.

7

Completing 'Voices' Jigsaw Puzzles
Jeanette Woolthuis

This chapter is about hearing voices and what you can do about it – and that is more than you would think. Voices are far more normal than everybody believes. Voices are not much stranger than real people or stranger than your own thoughts. In fact, it is strange that not everybody has heard voices at some point. However, people do get upset about voices, they find them weird, scary or dangerous; and if, as a child, you suddenly start hearing voices, adults start interfering with you. They are concerned, send you to a therapist – and what happens next ...?

A BIT OF A STRANGE JOB

I work as a therapist in my own practice. I prefer to work with children hearing voices. There was a time when I heard voices and I did not know how to deal with it. Now, I have learned how to do it and I do not hear voices any more – apart from when people talk to me, of course! After a while I decided to study to become a therapist. Initially I worked with children with all kinds of problems and also with adults for a while. Currently most children that come to me for therapy are voice hearers. I went on special courses for this, so that I understand the subject even better now. It is the best job in the world.

I will try and explain what I actually do in my job. Every therapist works in a different way. I will, therefore, just concentrate on my own work here. When you come to me for your first appointment, it means that you need help with something. For example, there is something that you cannot deal with or that bothers you. Some children are being bullied at school and they do not know how to stop this, others consider

themselves stupid and are afraid of doing anything wrong or they feel unhappy. Even when you hear voices that others cannot hear, you may need help. You (or your parents) will make an appointment and then we will meet. It is a good idea to meet first before you decide whether you want to go into therapy with me. You will talk about very personal things and that can be quite scary. That is why it is important, that there is a connection between us. It is you who, after all, chooses the therapy; if you do not want to come, there is not much point in coming to me, even if your parents want you to. Of course, you can agree a trial period with me, we will get to know each other and we can both decide whether we get on with each other or not.

AND WHAT DO WE DO NEXT?

When you start therapy with me, I will ask you many questions. In fact, an awful lot of questions, as I want to know exactly how you feel, who you are, what you are doing and I also want to know what your problems are. I will, therefore, also ask questions about the voices. Since I cannot feel what you feel, nor hear what your voices are saying, I need you to understand what you mean.

Sometimes the voices do not allow you to talk about them. However, I will still try and talk about them, you may be afraid of them – I am not! Sometimes I will agree on a certain sign with you; for instance, when the voices become too much of a bother and do not want you to talk about them any further. This is how I will still know what is happening to you.

We will also agree that you will tell me if there is something that you do not want to talk about, or cannot talk about (or simply do not know) or are not allowed to talk about. If you find talking difficult, I also work with drawings, usually the voices allow that, so that you do not have to talk. By drawing you can learn to talk! Sometimes I will talk to the voices too; for example, I may ask them whether they want to share their opinion on something or, if they become a real nuisance, I will ask them why they are doing that. Sometimes the voices want to talk to me and they will explain things. However, most of the time they suddenly go quiet then.

I also want to know whether you want to get rid of the voices or whether there are sweet voices that you want to keep on hearing. There are many children who hear kind voices too. If it does not bother you, you will not need therapy, since therapy is only useful when you have problems in your life or with your voices.

VOICES HAVE SOMETHING TO DO WITH YOU

Voices do not appear just for the fun of it. They talk to you or about you or about others, but you alone can hear them. That means they have something to do with you. Sometimes they are really nasty and they swear at you; sometimes they are nice and helpful. They can parrot you, sing, whisper, hum, scream or laugh at you. They can be nice and then suddenly turn nasty. Initially you may hear several voices and, at some point, fewer of them or vice versa; or you may hear noises for a while, followed by talking. Voices are just as varied as people, come in just as many different types and sounds. Sometimes they have names, sometimes you only recognise them by the way they speak. There are children that hear animals and things speak too. It can even happen that voices seem to hurt you. Since voices are different to everybody and they seem to say something about your life, I want to know exactly what they are saying and doing, even though you may find that very scary. Sometimes the voices can react badly and then you need the courage to talk about them anyway; but talking really helps! Sometimes the voices are so different from how you are that you do not want to have anything to do with them. However, we will still need to work out together why you have these voices.

YOUR CONTROL AND THE VOICES

If you hear voices that are punishing you if you do not do as they tell you or when you do something wrong, you can get pretty scared of them. Voices might threaten to let something bad happen to your parents or your brothers or sisters or they might threaten to kill your granny. Sometimes they threaten accidents, bad grades at school or they tell you that your friends never want to have anything to do with

you again. If you believe these voices and you are scared that they can really do these things, you are giving the voices a great deal of control. At the end of the day, voices do not have hands and feet in this world and, therefore, they can do nothing at all! However, sometimes it seems as if they have a lot of control and whatever they have threatened you with indeed happens. Together with you, I will find out how often the voices get it right and how it happened that they gained so much control over you. We will do all kinds of exercises at this point in order to regain your control again. Sometimes we do this through drawings, sometimes with role play. In the latter case, we will copy the voices and we will try and see whether you can react to them in a different way.

Some children feel real pain when the voices punish them. That can be quite a shock. I have never noticed that the voices are really able to do this. However, your body is able to fool you and the voices can, therefore, pretend to hurt you. I will try and explain how that can happen. Your body knows all kind of handy tricks. If you encounter something scary, you will get a shock. Your body will start doing all sorts of things; for example, producing adrenaline; a kind of super petrol which gives you super energy, allows you to run away fast and hardly feel any pain. This is very handy when, indeed, you need to act really quickly when something dangerous happens. However, if you have been scared for a long time such as when the voices truly scare you, your body will keep on pretending that you need to escape. You feel anxious, cold or, on the contrary, very hot; you feel nervous all over, or you are paralysed with fear. You may feel all kinds of strange tingling, stomach aches, headaches, tight chested, dizzy, have muscle problems or other things. The voices can make you believe that they are doing this to punish you. If you believe this, the voices gain more control, you become more scared and your body will react again. During therapy you will learn how to regain control and to be in charge of your own body and mind.

WHAT DOES IT ALL MEAN?

Without you realising it, voices say something about you. They talk in a certain way, with their own voice and they also behave in a certain way. When we talk about the voices, I will also ask you questions about everything you have been through and how you feel too. I will help

you understand why these voices are part of you and what they mean. I do not mean that you have to obey them when they set you very strange tasks, but that the voices are not there without a reason. Together we will look for similarities in your life. I will briefly explain what I mean here: the voices are concerned with something that happens or happened in your life. If you are very insecure and you are very scared to make a fool of yourself, the voices will be occupied with this too. Some voices will help you here, but other voices, on the contrary, will laugh at you. The voices will, in fact, tell you what you cannot cope with and what you are scared of. For example, when someone that you love very much has passed away, you will get very scared that you might lose even more people. At this point the voices might react by telling you that it is all your fault. They threaten to punish you when you are not nice enough to them or do not like it when you are angry. When you start talking about your fear, sadness and anger, voices cannot teach you anything any more and they will keep quiet.

COLIN

Colin is afraid of making mistakes at school. The three voices that he hears started talking to him when he had to do a presentation at school in front of his class and suddenly he did not know what to say any more. The class laughed at him and he was given a bad grade, because his teacher thought he had not prepared very well.

The voices tell him to do his very best and he is not allowed to score bad grades. The voices call him a lazy pig and tell him that he never does anything right. They continually compare him with someone else and tell him he is the biggest idiot on earth. They also threaten that they will tell his parents that he is a failure. The voices have made him believe that, as a punishment, he needs to go to a special children's home where he needs to stay until he has earned his freedom.

Colin makes more and more mistakes because he gets nervous and the teacher often tells him off. He does not do this on purpose, but the voices claim he does. When playing football, the voices laugh at him so much that he scores own goals by accident. All the spectators laugh at him or they are angry with him. His friends find he is becoming more and more of an idiot too. They do not want to be his friend any

longer. He is so upset now that he has told his parents that he is hearing voices. Together they are searching for help.

Initially it seemed as if the voices started with the bullying, but it turns out that Colin has three older brothers who are all very good at something. One can play the piano beautifully, one is becoming a professional football player and one is doing a degree and only gets high grades. Colin feels inferior. He is not really particularly good at anything. Everything is OK, but he does not have any special talents. Moreover, he is more than ten years younger than his brothers. He will never be able to overtake them. He is concerned that his parents do not find him clever enough, since they are always talking about his brothers and never about him. He cannot just pretend he is very good at something and being less clever than his brothers makes him very lonely and sad. He is stuck. The voices tell him exactly what the problem is. They bully him with the worst thing he can imagine: he is not good at anything.

BUT WHAT EXACTLY IS THERAPY?

Therapy is, in fact, like a puzzle, a jigsaw puzzle with hundreds of tiny pieces. It is like a jigsaw of which you still have all the pieces, but you have lost the picture, so that you do not know what the jigsaw will look like.

We will start off by discovering together what causes your problems. We will take all the pieces of the jigsaw out of the box and arrange them in their groups. First of all we will look for those pieces that form the edge; who are you, what you like and what you not like about yourself, what is your personality, what sort of things you do, who your friends are, your parents, siblings, how you are doing at school and what you have been through in your life and many more personal things about you. We will also look into the personal characteristics of the voices; who they are, or who they claim to be, what they are doing, when they present and when they don't, what makes them angry or satisfied, what they say, how they behave, when you hear them for the first time, who they resemble, etc.

We will then look for the jigsaw pieces that fit together immediately or the ones that you recognise immediately; sometimes they are in

the box pieced together already. We will put these down; they are done, we know that. For example, how you feel when the voices are talking, how much control you have and how much control the voices have, what you have already tried to counteract the voices, what works and what does not, whether you ever talk to other people about the voices and who you talk to about this, if the voices are right or if they talk nonsense, do you believe them or do you believe in their power, etc.

AND THAT IS WHEN THE REAL JIGSAW PUZZLE STARTS

Together we will look for pieces of the jigsaw that look similar; for instance, whether the voices sound like those of people you know or perhaps the voices are saying things about you that you agree with. It could also be that the behaviour of the voices is similar to something that has happened to you. In fact we are looking for connecting pieces, pieces of your life that resemble the things the voices are doing to you. Perhaps you felt very scared and powerless at some point in the past and you pretended at the time that everything was OK and now you are hearing voices that cause similar feelings. We will find out where these pieces fit until we get an idea of the overall picture of the jigsaw. That makes things far easier. This will clarify many things and they will become far less scary and threatening. Searching for pieces that look similar will still be quite a job, but we are getting an idea what the jigsaw should be looking like. You can even put the jigsaw away for a little while and continue later.

When making a real jigsaw you do not really discuss how you are piecing it together with each other. However, in therapy we will do that. I might ask you why you throw all the pieces back together in a heap in a fit of anger, when things do not seem to work out straightaway. Perhaps you are very scared that you cannot do anything right and everything always goes wrong. We will then discuss this and come up with plans which will teach you how to behave when you make mistakes (for example, dealing with fear of failure).

TOM

Tom sees himself as a bit of a softie, he says that he is not very macho and always scared. Together we will work out whether that is true and why he needs to be different from how he is. He also tells me that, at school, they bully him as the children in his class think it is dumb that he plays the violin and does not get involved in any sports like the others. Tom does not play football during the breaks, since he is not good at it and he is scared of falling over and hurting himself. The voices that he hears call him a softie and they swear at him. They agree with his classmates.

Together we come up with macho ways to stop the bullying by his classmates. He joins a judo club and he learns what, indeed, he can do with his body. At school he proves that he is strong and even that he can play football. He also dares to do a great deal more and he is not that scared of making a fool of himself any more. The voices suddenly do not find him a softie any more, because they notice that he is not scared any longer and that he can even get angry at them. In the end, the voices stop and he has not heard them since.

Handy tricks

So, you need some tricks in order to do well with the jigsaw. You will learn these tricks in therapy. Looking for the edges first is one of these tricks. It will give the jigsaw more structure and it does not become a mess. I will help you discover the tricks you already know. Together we will discover which tricks you have not tried yet. Sometimes we may try some out immediately and sometimes I may ask you to practice some at home or at school. Sometimes I come up with these tricks, sometimes it is you. We will look for those tricks that suit you best. These are, of course, no ordinary tricks. These are ways in which you deal with your life. For example, what to do when you feel bad, angry or sad. It is also about how you behave towards others, how you think about yourself or how you feel when you are doing something wrong. It is also about how you make friends or how you argue with people.

If you do not know how to do things or you do them in the wrong way, you will run into problems. For example, you may get very angry

because your mother is ill and she is very curt with you because she feels bad, but you do not allow yourself to be angry with her, because you feel so sorry for her and everyone wants you to be nice. So, instead of being angry, you are very nice as otherwise you feel guilty. The anger does not go away, but causes you to be angry with yourself. I will teach you to simply be angry and I will also teach you tricks to deal with your feeling of guilt.

With Colin we worked out whether the voices were perhaps saying things he was thinking himself – whether it was really true that he could be the most stupid boy on Earth. We talked about his brothers and how difficult it is to be the Benjamin who is last at everything. Together we explained to Colin's parents that he very much wants to hear from them that he is good too and, more than anything, that they show this to him. At the end of the day, he is unique too since he hears voices that can help him with his problems, whereas his brothers were never able to do this. Colin was finally able to get angry with his parents without being scared of being sent away. They made it very clear that they would never want to lose him and definitely not send him to a children's home. It took a while, but now Colin does not feel that worthless any more and he realises that other children make as many mistakes as he does. He has found his special talent after all; he is able to empathise with children who feel bad and helps them talk about it.

In this way you really learn how to complete a jigsaw. If, at a later date, you experience bad things again, at least, by then, you know a lot of tricks and you can come up with new solutions yourself. You do not need me or another therapist any more as, by then, you know what to do yourself. Hearing voices is not an additional, difficult problem or a hopeless case. If you are hearing voices and you learn to understand what is happening, you can regain control and lead your own life again.

Of course, you will also learn all kinds of tricks against the voices themselves. There are many ways in which you can deal with the voices. We will work out which ones you can practise and then we will try and think of new things. Many tricks have been thought out by voice hearers. However, every time I meet new children I learn new tricks from them.

AND HOW DO I DO THIS THERAPY?

I work in different ways:

- talking to you about things that bother you
- creative ways, like sculpting or painting
- physical ways, like relaxation exercises
- games, such as role play and drama
- writing exercises, like creating stories
- special drawing tasks
- homework tasks, like writing down when the voices are at their worst.

What I do very much depends on how you are doing and what suits you best. Sometimes I work in different ways with you, sometimes we just talk.

Handy tricks

- Voices are yours and voices do not own you.
- Voices do not have hands and feet, they cannot do anything to you.
- Voices get worse when you move in the right direction, they test how strong you have grown.
- You can be in control, though you may not always know how.
- Everything will come to an end, even unpleasant things.
- Talking about things helps, even if it is not allowed.
- Everybody has just as much chance to learn how to deal with it, you too.
- You are not the only one hearing voices.
- Everything can change.
- Are the voices always right or … ?
- Only scared voices threaten, what are they scared of?
- You are just as clever as the voices, so you can deal with them.
- You do not have to listen, you do not have to obey, they do not control you.

Jeannette Woolthuis has been active in the Dutch Patients Society for a number of years, as well as being a board member of 'Resonance', the Dutch Hearing Voices Network. She now has her own practice as a therapist for people who hear voices and specialises in working with children.

8

Young People Hearing Voices and Trauma

Our interest in children and young people hearing voices was stimulated by our studies on adults, where we found that about ten per cent started to hear voices in childhood. In the literature hallucinations or hearing voices by children and adolescents is mostly studied in the context of a variety of psychiatric states, such as schizophrenia (Bettes & Walker, 1987; Green et al., 1992; Galdos et al., 1993; Galdos & van Os, 1995), symptoms of anxiety and depression (Chambers et al., 1982; Garralda, 1984; Ryan et al., 1987), migraine (Schreier, 1998), trauma, dissociative processes and reactive psychosis (Famularo, 1992; Putman & Peterson, 1994; Altmann et al., 1997). All these studies concern selected clinical samples in which diagnostic procedures play an important role. Relatively little attention is given to the experience itself, the course and influence of events in the life history. In our studies on adults, we found in 70 per cent a relation between trauma and the onset of hallucinations. This made us wonder if, in children, there would also be a relationship between voices and events in the life history. We conducted a three-year follow-up study for which 80 children and adolescents were recruited between 8 and 18 years of age; about 50 per cent of which were in professional mental healthcare because of the voices. They were interviewed four times, with about one year in between the interviews.

METHODS, RESEARCH INSTRUMENTS AND PROCEDURES

In order to recruit children and adolescents who were hearing voices, extensive media contacts, formed in the course of a prior investigation were used (Romme & Escher, 1992).

In the research five instruments were used. The main instrument for our research was the *Maastricht Voices Interview for Children*, containing 12 sections. This interview consisted of the *Maastricht Voices Interview for Adults* (Romme, 1996; Romme & Escher, 1996) that we adapted for children with the aid of a clinical child psychologist. For general and specific psychopathology the Extended Brief Psychiatric Rating Scale (BPRS; Overall & Gorham, 1962; Lukoff et al., 1986) was assessed. As dissociation might be a reaction to trauma, we used the Dissociative Experience Scale (DES; Bernstein & Putman, 1986). With the Youth Self Report/11–18 (YSR) we measured general problem behaviour expressed as the total score (Verhulst et al., 1996) and, for the global level of functioning, the Children's Global Assessment Scale (CGAS; Shaffer et al., 1983) was used.

Nearly all of the subjects were interviewed at home. During the interviews, care was taken to elicit and record their experiences, rather than those of their parents. At the end of each interview, research staff made a report covering all the data collected. This was subsequently discussed with the research team, in order to discuss problems and ambiguities and to create continuing consensus on how to conduct the interview and rate answers in a standardised way.

One of the sections of this interview concerns a total score of life events that might be related to the onset of the voices. In a structured way, about 22 childhood events/trauma that in the pilot-study children related to the onset of voice hearing were scored 'present' or 'absent' (for example, death, illness, accidents, friends moving away, changing school, first menstruation, pregnancy, unrequited love, arguments, parental divorce, repeating school year, other life events, etc.). The last question being if the child thought there was a relationship between the onset of the voices and the life event mentioned. In another section, receipt of professional help and help-seeking behaviour was assessed by asking whether professional help was being received in relation to the voices, and/or what kind of care in relation to the voices was received.

ANALYSIS

The mean age was 12.9 years (SD = 3.1; range 8–19 years). Around half (53.8 per cent) were female. We found no gender-related significance. About 50 per cent of the children were in professional mental healthcare because of the voices. Not being in care did not mean that the voices were not problematic. In the first year, 70 per cent of the children had problems at home and 82 per cent at school because of the voices (Escher & Romme, 1998).

The rate of voice discontinuation was 25.3, 26.0 and 47.7 per cent at respectively the one-, two- and three-year follow-up interview. The cumulative incidence of voice discontinuation was 60 per cent. Voice reoccurrence was 13 per cent (*N* = 4). Voices remained in subjects with higher ratings on BPRS anxiety, depression and hallucinations and in those with high frequency of voice hearing. Voice persistence was also associated with a high scores on the DES, older age and lack of clear triggers in time and place (Escher et al., 2002a). Thirteen children (16 per cent) displayed evidence of delusional ideation over at least one of the three follow-up periods, of which seven (nine per cent) had begun again.

In order to examine whether the effect of predictors of voice discontinuation varied as a function of being in care or being a 'case' in terms of high levels of psychopathology, problem behaviour or low levels of social functioning, we fitted interactions between predictors on the one hand and receipt of mental healthcare, 'case' level of psychopathology (defined as score greater than 90th percentile on BPRS sum score), 'case' level of problem behaviour (score greater than 90th percentile on the YSR) and 'case' level of poor social functioning (score greater than 90th percentile on the CGAF) on the other. Having mental healthcare in itself did not influence the probability of voice discontinuation.

A high trauma score was found. Of the children, 86.3 per cent reported one or more traumas around the time of the onset of the hallucinations.

TRAUMA

Most children, who reported trauma, experienced one trauma (48 per cent). Two traumas were reported by 15.9 per cent and three by 7.3 per cent. We distinguished six groups of trauma: confrontation with death; problems in and around home; problems in and around school; physical condition interfering with development; traumas in relation to sexuality and a group of traumas that did not fit into the other groups. Children who experienced more trauma, more often looked for care.

	N	Total	%
Confrontation with death	18	18	22.5
Problems at home			
Serious tension with parents and or brothers/sisters	10		
Divorced parents	6		
Moving house	3	19	23.7
Problems around the school situation			
Ability problems	9		
Changing schools	7		
Being bullied	3	19	23.7
Physical condition interfering with development			
Brain damage caused by traffic accident	1		
A physical health problem with long-term hospital admission	4		
Birth trauma	2	7	8.7
In relation to sexuality			
Sexual abuse *	4		
Rejection in love	1		
Abortion	1	6	6.2
Other kinds of trauma/problems			
Seeing something weird	3		
Anaesthesia	1	4	4.8
No trauma	11	11	13.7

*The small number of reported sexual abuses might be related to the research context. Most children and adolescents came to participate in this research through their parents. The four girls who reported sexual abuse were not abused by parents or siblings, but by people they knew — like the boy next door, classmates, a boyfriend and an uncle.

Although one or more traumas might have happened around the time of the onset, for most children the relation between the onset and their voices was not clear. For 11.2 per cent, there was no relation at all; 26.2 per cent reported a relation, but most children (62.6 per cent) did not connect the voices to a traumatic experience. For them, there was no relationship between the voices and themselves. During the research period we noticed that parents and children talked about and reflected the time the voices started, specially when the characteristics of the voices were indicative of the problems that lay at the root; like in a simple example, the boy who heard the voice of his teacher who was very abusive, or children who heard the voice of a dead grandparent. Voices could be metaphoric in cases of ability problems. When the children changed schools and the voices disappeared, parents and children then realised the relationship.

Some children did not mention any kind of trauma in the first interview, but did so in the second or third. For example, a girl of 18 had a total DES score of 60 at the first interview. She reported no trauma. At the second interview, being admitted to a psychiatric hospital and diagnosed as schizophrenic, this girl told the interviewer about the sexual abuse when she was 12. She then had a boyfriend of 19. The boyfriend gave her drugs and let his friends sexually abuse her in this condition. She did not tell anyone and asked the interviewer not to tell her parents or therapist, as she felt ashamed of what had happened and guilty rather than traumatised.

VOICES AND DEVELOPMENT

Having professional mental healthcare is not related to discontinuation of the voices. However, during the interviews it became evident that a number of children changed. They made more friends and life seemed

to be broader than the voices. As some children stated: 'There is more to life than my voices.' With other children, the initial problems, often relating to the onset of the voices, were not solved and seemed, still, to influence their life. These changes seemed to concern development. It looked as if development had a positive influence on the discontinuation of the voices. We, therefore, became interested in development and the relation between discontinuation or continuation.

To assess the quality of the child's development we developed our own instrument. To avoid stigmatising statements about development, we documented changes that had been discussed during the three-year follow-up. Using a grounded theory approach (Glaser & Strauss, 1967), we attempted to assume a naïve position with regard to relevant factors for developmental outcome and its relationship to treatments. We did not originally hypothesise the issues that might arise; they emerged during the follow-up period. In following a grounded theory approach we thought that it would be sensible to include the issues about the relationship of continuation or discontinuation of voices and development of the child in our report. Using grounded theory method-ology was also appropriate because of our search for knowledge in a meagrely researched field of inquiry.

Prior to analysing any data and blind to possible relations we specified our criteria for undisturbed development, based on discussion within the research team of what was observable and measurable in the developmental process:

1. acquiring more friends at the peer group level
2. knowing better what they wanted to become in life
3. learning to cope better with emotions
4. having fewer conflicts within the family and at school
5. a positive report on development reported by the child concerned and/or by the parents

For each child a conclusion was made in terms of: a negative change; undisturbed development/disturbed development or no change between baseline and last interview. When four out of five elements were positive, then positive development was marked. In the analysis we included only the 68 children who participated throughout the

whole research period. Outcome factors are the discontinuation of the voices as well as the development of the child.

There is a significant association between discontinuation of the voices and positive development ($X^2(1) = 18.56$, P <. 001). However, discontinuation of the voices does not always result in positive development. From the 45 children with discontinuation, 38 (84 per cent) showed a positive and seven had a negative development.

Equally so, continuation of the voices does not always result in negative development. Out of the 22 children who still heard voices, negative development is seen in seven children in professional care. In the 22 children who continued to hear voices, negative development was seen in 15 (68 per cent).

	N	Continuation of hearing voices		Discontinuation of hearing voices	
		Positive development	Negative development	Positive development	Negative development
Professional care	39	3	10	19	7
No care	29	4	5	19	1
Total	68	7	15	38	8

If professional mental healthcare is not related to discontinuation of voices but development is, this suggests that development might be of a greater importance for overcoming the distress of voices. This points out the signal functions of the voices.

CONCLUSIONS

Although the outcome of the research showed that hearing voices in itself is not a continuous phenomenon, and that the possibility that voices might disappear is quite high (60 per cent), it would be more profitable to look at hearing voices as a signal of problems in the ongoing

life history than to identify the voices as a symptom of an illness or a defect and reduce, thereby, the meaning of the experience. This idea is supported by the high number of traumas reported at the onset of voice hearing.

This point of view also explains the great diversity between individuals concerning the content, the triggers and the problems relating to the onset of the voice hearing. This also explains why all theories arising from research that identify hearing voices with psychopathology do not explain the phenomenon satisfactorily.

As a conclusion we propose that voices are seen as a human characteristic and an indication of problems that need to be solved, instead of a psycho-pathological phenomenon. Explained in this way it is understandable that there is no contradiction between patients and non-patients. Promoting development by compensating or by solving the initial problem is, in this way of reasoning, also more effective than blaming the hallucinations and trying to suppress them.

9

Voice Collective:
Learning from parents who've been there
Rachel Waddingham

Voice Collective is a London-wide project to develop peer support opportunities for young people who hear, see or sense things that others don't. Launched by Mind in Camden in April 2009, the project has changed over the past year to respond to an overwhelming level of need. In addition to working with young people themselves, we've formed alliances with parents, carers, teachers, youth workers and a range of other professionals to help them understand and support those struggling with the voices they hear.

Our first contact with families is often an email or phone call from a parent who is feeling isolated, extremely worried for their child's wellbeing and under pressure to find the best support possible for them. Whilst some have good relationships with the mental health services, others have expressed real confusion and concern at what they feel is a lack of options and support on offer. Navigating the child and adolescent mental health services can be a bit like entering a maze blindfolded without a guide. Thankfully, as well as providing some support for their child, we have been able to act as that guide (or help them find someone who can).

It's testament to the tenacity and determination of parents that they, rather than professionals, were the first to seek out the Voice Collective project for their children. These parents were eager to embrace a more hopeful and positive view of their child's experiences and instinctively see the benefit in peer support to facilitate this.

One unique aspect to our project is that both the development worker and myself have personal experience of voices or visions to draw on. Parents and young people have sometimes found it helpful to meet

with us in person, whether or not they eventually access the group. Neither of us sees ourselves as a role model. My own journey has been a rocky one and I sincerely hope that those with whom we work follow an easier path. Still, we are living proof that it is possible to live, work and enjoy life whether or not you hear voices. Once you know how to deal with them, voices are not a barrier to living the life you choose.

This chapter has given us a welcome opportunity to share some of the experiences of the parents we have supported, both positive and negative. It is our hope that within these pages you will recognise something of use to your own situation. It's good to know that others tread similar paths to you. As you'll already know through reading this book, your child is not alone in hearing voices. It stands to reason, then, that as a parent or supporter you're in good company too.

SIDESTEP THE BLAME GAME

Guilt is a destructive emotion.

In your search to make sense of what is happening, it's all too easy to fall prey to self-blame. Some of the parents we meet have spent countless hours examining their actions with a fine-tooth comb, looking for answers in all the things they did and didn't do.

Whilst we encourage parents to think about what the voices might be saying about problems their child is experiencing, there is simply nothing to be gained from being consumed with guilt or self-recrimination. Without exception, it has been obvious to us how much the parents we meet love and cherish their children. Never lose sight of this in yourself.

CHOOSE YOUR ADVISORS CAREFULLY

What wasn't so helpful was random surfing on the net. It kind of overwhelmed me with the statistics and data on voices, and the dire predictions.

If your child is hearing or seeing things it's natural to want to understand more about what they are experiencing. Many parents spend considerable time and energy searching for answers using the Internet;

others seek advice from medical, spiritual or trusted others. The challenge here is that there is no single way of viewing voices. Ask 100 experts and you may well get 100 different opinions. Even research itself is not unaffected by the values of the person conducting it.

We all have our own perspective and this will always influence any advice or suggestions we give. At the end of the day, it is you and your child who live with their experiences 24/7. It's important that you listen critically to information and advice and avoid taking it at face value. Use your experience thus far to make an informed choice about whether or not other people's ideas are helpful.

ASK THE RIGHT QUESTIONS

Follow your instincts and remember you know your child better than anyone else.

If your child begins to hear or see things that distress them, the first question many parents ask is: 'WHY?' The sheer range of ideas around why people hear voices can be dizzying and you might find yourself tying yourself in knots trying, seeking the clarity that expert opinion and diagnoses appear to promise. In my experience, it can be more helpful to change your focus. There are lots of questions you can ask that will give you real and practical clues about what is going on for your child and how to best support them.

You can ask:

- Why is my child hearing these particular voices and at this particular time?
- What do they tell me about how my child is feeling right now?
- What is happening in their life that they find difficult?
- What exactly is it about the voices or visions that is causing my child a problem?
- When is it less intense and easier to cope with?
- Are the voice or visions the source of the distress, or are they playing a role in helping them cope with something else?

This isn't about becoming your child's therapist; if they're struggling to cope it's best to find someone with specialist skills in this area to help them work it through. It's simply about gaining confidence in your skills and abilities as a parent to treat the voices or visions as you would any emotional problem your child may be having. Trust your instincts, engage with your child's experiences and listen to what they tell you. All the important answers are there to be found together.

KEEP YOUR TOOLBOX TOPPED UP

Give comfort after a particularly unpleasant experience – a cuddle, a cup of tea – whatever seems right at the time.

As a parent, you'll already have a range of tools that help you to support your child's wellbeing. Hugs, creativity, listening, staying grounded, routine, flexibility, comfort, distraction, healthy eating, creating a safe space – all of these are equally helpful if your child is struggling to cope with their voices or visions.

I need to contact others who have worked with this before, so that I know what steps to follow and how to give him the best care I can.

On top of this, there are a plenty of tips, tricks and strategies that you can learn to deal with particularly scary or distressing experiences. Be active in seeking these out. After all, the more tools you have in your toolbox the more confident you will be in your ability to help your child cope on a day-to-day basis. Don't forget that you're not the only person to be in this situation, so you don't need to reinvent the wheel. Get ideas by listening to people who can cope with the voices they hear, those who support them and the Voice Collective website.

I acknowledge that what she hears is real to her. Remind her where she is and that she is safe.

As a starting point, we've found grounding and relaxation techniques really helpful. Feeling safe is a great foundation to build on. Strategies that help build young people's confidence, self-esteem and assertiveness are invaluable too.

Ask them how they feel and what they think might be helpful.

When given the opportunity, children and young people can develop really inventive ways of coping that are unique to their own situation. Try to encourage a practical problem-solving approach and help them take control of their experience. Voices or visions only have the power that we give them, no matter how scary they appear to be.

FOCUS ON THEIR STRENGTHS AND ABILITIES

My daughter is stronger than I ever realised – I'm proud of her.

If your child is struggling, it's easy for everyone around them to lose sight of the young person's strength and resources. Often the young people we meet have lost sight of these too and need help to recognise, and develop, them. No matter how difficult the situation, I have never failed to be impressed by the resilience of the young people at Voice Collective.

If you find yourself falling into the trap of seeing, and talking about, your child in terms of their problems, it can really help to actively look for the positives. What have they got going for them? What do you like to do together? Can any of their vulnerabilities be seen as a potential strength? What do you admire about them? Try viewing your child through a different lens.

This in no way means that you should ignore, disregard or dismiss the problems that your child faces. It's simply a way of approaching these issues from a different angle. Once recognised, your child's strengths can be built on and used to help them cope with the more difficult aspects of their experience. More than this, your faith in them and the hope you carry with you will help them to keep hold of it themselves.

DON'T GO IT ALONE

Never be afraid to ask for advice, support and help.

Everyone needs a support network. In an ideal world, we'd all have a range of different people able to help out in different ways. Some of

the parents we have met are extremely well supported by their partners, families and friends and understand what outside agencies can do to help.

Unfortunately this experience is not universal. Some parents we meet feel extremely isolated and under immense pressure to provide everything their child and family needs. This often happens when they feel let down by the support offered to them, or are simply unaware of what's out there.

Explore all *options of support both for you and your child, such as Voice Collective – who can not only relate to what your child is experiencing, but can provide effective and empathic support for both your child and you.*

No matter how isolated you feel, there are people out there who are willing to help. The trick is to find out what's available in your area and how to access it. Other than Voice Collective, contacting Young Minds is a good first step. They run an excellent parents' helpline which is intended to both provide emotional support and help you link in with services that can help on a more ongoing basis.

At Voice Collective we're currently developing a peer support group for parents. We hope that this will provide them with a much-needed space to offload, support one another and keep hold of the positives. If you live in or around London, contact us for more information about this. If not, you could always speak to a local carers' or parents' organisation to see if you could start something in your area. Some of the best initiatives start from people recognising a need for something new and joining together to meet it.

GETTING THE BEST OUT OF THE CHILD AND ADOLESCENT MENTAL HEALTH SERVICES

I have always called for support and advice from my daughter's teams when I've felt out of my depth and also when I know she needs more support than I am able to provide.

If your child is struggling to cope, you may be referred to the child and adolescent mental health services (CAMHS) or an Early Intervention in

Psychosis team (EIP). Our experience of CAMHS and EIP teams has been largely positive. We have excellent working relationships with a number of teams and I'm encouraged by their flexible approach to understanding distressed children and young people. If you have a good relationship with these teams, they can be an invaluable resource.

Being involved in decision making by various professionals also helped.

Unfortunately we have met some parents who have felt disappointed or frustrated by their contact with the mental health services. When problems occur, they seem to centre around three core issues: lack of choice; feeling excluded from decision-making; professionals and parents having a completely different, and incompatible, understanding of the situation. These problems have sometimes led to breakdowns in communication that leave the parents feeling even more isolated and confused.

It seems within the Mental Health system in the UK there is little available for children who hear voices. When I questioned this lack of support for my daughter, I was labelled as uncooperative/obstructive.

If you feel this is happening to you, or you are concerned about any aspect of your child's care, seek out an advocacy service to help you raise this in a positive way. Advocates are experts in navigating situations like these and will work alongside you to find a solution. They specialise in helping people get their point of view heard and can make invaluable allies.

The CBT delivered by the psychologist was excellent and made a huge difference during the short time that it lasted.

Psychological therapies, including art therapy, counselling and cognitive behavioural therapy, are often welcomed by the young people we have met. They provide a space where your child feels heard and is supported to work through their distress. Unfortunately, provision of these is not yet universal so some families have had to be very active in pushing for them. If you, or your child, want to look at your full range of options, speak to people in the know. Young Minds and local advocacy services are experts in this field and can be your guide.

FIND THE BALANCE FOR YOU AND YOUR CHILD

Listen to your child and take them seriously, but don't forget to look after yourself too.

As Sandra has said elsewhere, it's important that the voices and visions don't become the centre of your lives. If these experiences distress your child, however, it is easier said than done. Balance is key, but can be hard to find when you feel under pressure.

Parents have told us how they feel it's important to accept the reality of their child's voice-hearing experience, whilst not letting it become the only topic of conversation. Children and young people need encouragement to be just that – young. They need space to have hopes, fears, worries, dreams, arguments, sulks, anxieties and dramas above and beyond the voices or visions.

You, as a parent, need to find that balance too. When I was struggling with voices and paranoia, my parents – realising their every conversation was dominated by their concern for me – implemented a 'no Rachel-talk after 8pm' rule. It was a stroke of genius. Remember to focus on your needs too – whether it's nurturing a romantic relationship or friendship, renewing an old hobby, studying something that interests you or just taking time to relax.

Without exception, all of the young people with whom I've worked have felt worried about the impact that their distress is having on their family. Keeping yourself healthy will help them stay healthy too.

USEFUL RESOURCES FOR PARENTS AND SUPPORTERS

Voice Collective
W: www.voicecollective.co.uk
T: 020 7625 9042
E: info@voicecollective.co.uk

Young Minds
W: www.youngminds.org.uk
T: 020 7336 8445 (office), 0808 802 5544 (parents' helpline)

National Youth Advocacy Service
W: www.nyas.net
T: 0800 616101 (helpline)
E: help@nyas.ne

Parentline Plus
W: www.parentlineplus.org.uk
T: 0808 800 2222 (24/7 helpline)

Rachel Waddingham has heard voices and seen visions since her youth. After almost losing herself in the mental health system during her 20s, she feels lucky to have heard Romme and Escher's message of hope and understanding through the Hearing Voices Network. Rachel now works at Mind in Camden as the manager of Voice Collective, a London-wide peer support project for young people who hear, see or sense things others don't. She is continually humbled by the strength and openness of those she works with and would like to thank them for their help in shaping this chapter.

10

'Resonance Association' Advice for Parents
Thea Boom-Legierse

When your child indicates that he/she is hearing voices, a lot is happening. Every parent's innermost desire is to have a happy and cheerful child who travels through life without any complications. When a child starts to hear voices, initially parents will not recognise the problems, nor will they accept this to be something that is part of their child. It is a natural reaction to deny everything and to be just as flexible as children can be in terms of finding all kinds of ways to continue as normal for the sake of love, and peace and quiet, and to simply accept the unaccountable behaviour of the child. Sometimes, some signals are needed such as from school to wake up the parents.

From the moment my son told me he was hearing voices, I understood that many of his unexplained problems and moods had been caused by his voice hearing. He did not sleep well, had tantrums in which I did not recognise him at all, had difficulty concentrating, wanted to die sometimes, had head- and stomach ache attacks without physical cause. I was very shocked and could foresee a psychiatric hospital admission in later life.

I searched for and found help for him as well as good support for myself. I was given advice via the Stichting Weerklank ('Resonance Association') in the Netherlands and I learned a great deal from the contacts with voice hearers within the carers' network. Furthermore, there is some wonderful literature about this subject from all points of view. Reading and gaining more in-depth knowledge has helped me as a parent. It was difficult not to make his problems mine too.

For many years I gave parents advice over the telephone as a volunteer for the association, Resonance. This is where I realised how important information can be for parents.

WHAT DID I TELL PARENTS WHO PHONED US?

Until the age of eight it is very normal for children to have invisible friends. Parents should not be concerned about this at all. Children are highly sensitive personalities. They feel and experience things at another level compared to us adults. Some of us will keep this sensitivity for the rest of our lives and can benefit from this. Unfortunately hearing or even seeing things that others do not see or hear does not always make life easier.

If parents are getting worried, they start to wonder where to get help. When does voice hearing need help? On the basis of my own experiences and from the experience I gained from the telephone service I ran for the Resonance Association for many years, I drew up the following list. This list is certainly not complete, but provides an indication, if:

- your child looks unhappy
- there are fears and unexplained tantrums
- your child does not sleep well
- your child often suffers from headaches or stomach aches without physical causes
- there are concentration problems
- you find that your child suffers from extreme fear of failure
- you sometimes do not recognise your own child, in his or her behaviour

WHAT CAN YOU DO?

First of all, always accept your child and be prepared to believe what you are told. Children who hear voices are very sensitive and, by rejecting them, it is more likely that you will lead them to isolation than a solution. Secondly, you are the one who offers structure to their lives where they are not able to do this themselves. They really need structure just as much as peace, security and simplicity. There are often too many stimuli around them. Television and computers suck up energy, mobile phones influence our complete energy system. All of these technological developments mean progress, but at the

same time they are factors that burden our nervous system.

Moreover, children hearing voices have an overactive nervous system anyway. These children benefit from attention, 'earthing'. With earthing I literally mean something that will bring them back down to earth. They live in their head. Images and/or thoughts or voices pull them away from daily life. That is very tiring. Parents can get them back being involved in daily life again by letting them feel and see things again. Voices and the 'other spheres' or other reality can have an immense influence and you are the perfect person to create clarity in their world.

PARENTS SEARCHING FOR HELP AND ASKING FOR ADVICE

For children who hear voices the following are very important:

- order/structure in everything
- being outside a lot, preferably walking in the countryside; this is grounding
- a good diet, with few additives
- clearly defined mealtimes
- five eating times with sufficient vegetables and fruit or nuts can be really good
- limit soft drinks with colour additives
- no synthetic clothes
- as few stress-triggering factors as possible. Too many activities, even though they may seem like relaxation (sport), can lead to overload
- avoid busy shopping centres, cinemas, amusement or theme parks etc. and, if possible, public transport
- a good day and night rhythm. Fixed bed or rest times, particularly when sleeping is a problem
- touch, e.g., foot massage can bring them back into their body from the head. Just sitting together for a while or stroking from the head down the back
- set times for TV and computer
- no mobile telephone

- friends can be tiring, let them choose for themselves when they feel or do not feel like socialising
- as a parent be alert about signals of overload; like crying, nagging, compulsion or sleeplessness
- try to avoid things escalating. This is not easy as you should not become a parent giving in to everything for the sake of keeping the peace. This does not help setting boundaries, the structure that they need so desperately
- be creative and always stay smart

Tips for relaxing

- bath with lavender, lime blossom or St John's Wort oil, water provides peace and relaxation, a lovely long shower can be helpful too
- foot massage with lavender or St John's Wort oil
- hands in the earth, e.g., gardening
- sea and sand, or trees, if they are nearby, provide enormous feelings of well-being, as does most contact with nature
- exercise, without it being result-driven to encourage deep breathing
- reading to them
- letting them draw, paint, chalk, mould things. Let them model their voices or their emotions. With an image or a sculpture, they can decide for themselves what they want to do with it. The voices manipulate them, now they can manipulate the voices. Allow space for their creativity, ideally with natural materials
- listen to their stories without any form of judgement. Set a specific amount of time that you will spend with them and inform them of this. This is how they will learn to set limits to listening to their voices too
- teach them to say no to the voices, to make choices, to make them feel more important than the voices
- confirm their positivity
- just stick to a small world
- a good diet is essential for voice hearers. One thing can be healthy for one and a burden for others; consult a dietician for advice

- children who hear voices often react well to herbs, e.g., lemon balm tea or lime blossom tea in the late afternoon or early evening can help sleeping and provide relaxation
- alternative remedies can help, but these need therapeutic guidance

Children can be signposts for their parents. Children hearing voices often occupy a special place because of their sometimes highly sensitive nature. This asks for adjustment and fine-tuning. As a parent of a very special human being I wish you all wisdom in your path to being a good guide.

I learned a great deal from my voice-hearing child. He showed me a direction for my life, which I probably would not have found otherwise. I learned a lot from my voluntary work at the Resonance Association, where I was involved in the telephone service advising other parents.

My son is 24 now and he has recently started to live on his own. As a mother, I do not have any influence at all on his life any more. I cannot exert any influence in stress situations and the circumstances that may trigger these. This is 'letting-go' and I trust that he, with his emotionally vulnerable personality, will find his way.

Prayer

God grant me the serenity to accept things I cannot change,
Courage to change things I can, and
The wisdom to know the difference.

11

Parents' Experiences
Anne, Marie Louise and Karin

ANNE'S STORY

In an email to Sandra Escher Anne wrote: When Hannah was about six or seven years old, she told me about a voice she heard. She was absolutely adamant that the voice was not her own thoughts and definitely not an 'imaginary' friend. I qualified in 1985 as a mental health nurse, and so my first thoughts were of childhood schizophrenia. Then I attended one of the first workshops you presented at UCE (the University of Central England in Birmingham), and learned a lot about childhood voice hearers. I was lucky to speak with you at the end of the workshop and asked your advice about how I could help Hannah. Your advice was absolutely great. You told me that the best thing I could do was to relax, not become stressed about this, listen to my daughter and accept the voice as a normal event for her.

From this I was able to talk with Hannah about the voice and we decided to call him 'Mike'. Sometimes Mike was funny and made her laugh, but at times (usually when Hannah was tired or stressed at school) he could be very nasty and made her upset. On a few occasions Hannah woke in the middle of the night and became very distressed by Mike. I tried using distraction, but this didn't really work, so I asked a colleague, who is a family therapist, if he could recommend any techniques. Nathan, my colleague, suggested finding out what Mike had said and turning it into a cartoon/joke, because if I could get Hannah laughing at Mike it would be difficult for her to feel frightened at the same time. This worked really well, and we dealt with Mike as the situation needed it. When Hannah got to be 11 years old I realised that

she had been talking less and less about Mike and hadn't mentioned him for about a year. So, I asked her whether she had heard from Mike recently. Her answer was 'Who's Mike?' She had forgotten all about him, and when I reminded her she said that she couldn't remember the last time she had heard him. Since then she has not heard any voices.

Your advice was really useful because it normalised the situation for me. Instead of seeing my daughter as being possibly mentally ill, I was able to see her as someone who was well, bright and had a quirky personality trait which made her an individual. Someone special rather than someone who needed professional input. Hannah has dyscalculia and some features of dyslexia. She has always been an avid reader, but has difficulty in handling some aspects of mathematics. Learning times tables (two twos are four, three twos are six, etc.) was a nightmare for her. Also, she has some short-term memory problems. So, if I ask her to do three chores in the house she will do the third one, she may be able to remember the second one, but the first chore will be forgotten. We have developed strategies for this, like writing things down and, when she was younger, I set fairly rigid routines for times like bedtime, getting ready for school, etc. She is 15 years old now, and so bedtimes are not really an issue any more. However, when Hannah was younger she coped with the dyscalculia by concentrating really hard at school, so when I picked her up she would usually be very tired. I think this was a factor in determining when Hannah heard her voice.

Hannah is now studying for GCSE examinations and is predicted to get mostly A and B grades. She is far more motivated than I was when I was at school, and is top of her year in physics. You will have to excuse my boasting about her; I don't often get the opportunity!

Incidentally, when Hannah was about eight or nine years old, I was discussing her progress at school with her headteacher, and I told the headteacher that Hannah was a voice hearer. The headteacher immediately became very concerned and started trying to organise an appointment with an educational psychologist. I refused for a number of reasons. First, I felt that Hannah was getting all the help she needed from her father and myself and any assessment by a psychologist would only serve to give her a psychiatric label. The headteacher was very unhappy about this and tried to push me into taking Hannah to see a

psychologist. In the end, I informed her that I had taken advice from one of the foremost leaders in the field of children who hear voices, and that I was happy that everything that Hannah needed was available within the family and was being carried out. Without your advice I would not have been able to be so assertive.

Anyway, I must finish now before this email develops into a book! I hope you found my experience interesting and, once again, thank you very, very much for your extremely helpful and positive advice. It was just what was needed.

MARIE LOUISE'S STORY

After a difficult time in my life I became pregnant with Tamsin. John and I already had two daughters (Jolanda and Holly) when we decided to take a 12-year-old foster child (Monique) into our family. This addition to our family was accompanied by many problems, since Monique had been through a lot and she even found normal things difficult. Dealing with and trusting other people around her were very difficult too. After a while, things did not work out any more and the Child Protection League put Monique into a children's home again. That was better for her and for us, but I felt empty, depressed but, most of all, sad.

When, following that, I got pregnant again, it felt like a present. We were very happy and we were looking forward to this new, little person so very much. The pregnancy went swimmingly and Tamsin was born on a beautiful, sunny Sunday. Tamsin was an easy, sweet, always happy and fun child. For Tamsin everything was fine and she enjoyed all the attention. As a toddler she made up a small imaginary crocodile. She took the little animal everywhere. We had to take care where we were sitting and standing as the crocodile was always there and, of course, we were not allowed to sit or stand on it. If she 'forgot' the little animal we had to go back and get it. She had this little crocodile in her life for a long time and even a visit to the zoo did not make her change her mind. Her crocodile was small, sweet and fitted into her little hand.

When Tamsin was six or seven years old I found out that she heard voices and I was very upset. Tamsin described the voices as follows: 'In my head it seems as if I am sitting in the middle of a small room with a

group of men who are angry with me!' The voices were always angry (never friendly) with Tamsin and made her insecure. To me that seemed very scary and difficult too. No wonder that Tamsin would be quiet then.

At first I did not do anything about it and I hoped that the voices would go away by themselves. After a couple of weeks we went to the doctor after all, the GP comforted me, I did not need to worry. The voices would disappear by themselves, like the little crocodile.

However, the voices remained! I found it very scary and did not dare to talk to anyone about it; I needed to come to terms with it first (and as long as I did not talk about it, the problem seemed smaller), but that was not easy. Fortunately Tamsin was not worried about it at all, as to her the voices were normal and she probably thought that everybody was hearing voices. She told her girlfriends about her voices in an open and honest way.

When Laura's parents (a friend of Tamsin), read an article about children hearing voices out loud, Laura thought that her parents were talking about Tamsin. The next day Laura's mother came to me with the article – if Laura thinks that this article is about Tamsin, you may want to read it. Indeed, it was certainly an article that I wanted to read and, more than that, the article has, for many years, given me the faith that everything will be alright with Tamsin again. Dr Sandra Escher and Prof Romme wrote about a study with children hearing voices and they approached voices as emotions that people had not come to terms with yet. For me, this was the first time I read such information, about hearing voices, where they did not link it to schizophrenia. Since I was pretty worried about Tamsin's voices, I regularly searched for information, but everything I found did not seem to apply to Tamsin and scared me. Despite the fact that I did not know what kind of an emotion Tamsin had not come to terms with, my intuition told me that this was the road I had to follow.

Tamsin regularly heard voices and became very quiet, adapted to the environment and tried to make herself as invisible as possible. She was a child who always adapted to her environment, therefore also to her voices and she never got angry. She adapted effortlessly to everything and everybody without it seeming to bother her. She was happy, friendly and cheerful.

In the third grade at primary school, all subjects went swimmingly,

it was just reading that she had not quite mastered yet. After a year of reading lessons, she was only able to read a few words. To me this was inexplicable as Tamsin was a smart child in every area, so why could she not read? The transition to grade 4 was a problem, but I agreed with the teacher that, during the summer holidays, I would read with Tamsin five minutes every day and after the holidays it would be decided in which grade Tamsin would continue. After six weeks of relaxing exercises, Tamsin was at the same reading level as her classmates. This was the first time I encountered Tamsin's strength and intelligence. In hindsight, I thought that during reading lessons at school Tamsin would be hearing voices as a result of which she could not or did not dare to concentrate on learning how to read. At home she was probably not disturbed by the voices and, therefore, she was able to learn how to read fast. Tamsin went through primary school as a normal child. She had many friends and could cope with the academic level. However, the voices remained.

When she noticed that some of her classmates did not understand her voices, she held a talk about voice hearing in the seventh grade. All children found this enormously interesting and found the voices normal (at least in Tamsin's case). She did not become the odd one out, she was simply Tamsin and she simply remained Tamsin.

Tamsin accepted the voices and she did not know any better, but I was concerned and kept an eye on her. I kept on looking for information and that did not make me any happier. Every time when things were not going well with Tamsin, I tried to protect her and looked for appropriate help. All the information that I found dealt with schizophrenia, psychoses and drugs which suppress emotions. I kept this information far away from Tamsin. For me, it was difficult to put all this information into perspective, but for a child not even 12 yet, it would have been far more difficult. Tamsin had to develop into a mature adult and she should not link all this information about voice hearers to herself and as a consequence become insecure or, even worse, to perceive herself as not normal and ill, as Tamsin is such a very sweet and normal person. At the same time I wanted to be honest with her and not paint an inaccurate picture as she heard voices and she needed to deal with them. However, she also had to learn to deal with the way in which other people reacted to voice hearers. Not everybody reacts

in a very understanding way. Most people are scared of it and have already made up their minds before they have even met the person in question.

All in all, I have tried to only give information to Tamsin that she could cope with at that particular time. Furthermore, I have encouraged her to be open and honest about her voices and I told that she should not feel embarrassed about it. Some people have bent legs and Tamsin has voices. However, whenever things were not going well for Tamsin, I would try and seek help and I would just go with my instincts. I very much wanted someone to tell me that we were doing the right things. Tamsin was still so young and what about when she gets to puberty, will I still be able to help her then? All in all, Tamsin needed help and I needed help too. We tried different ways, but whenever I did not have a good feeling about it, I took Tamsin by the hand again and left.

When Tamsin was about ten years old, things were going well for her. I was worried that things would be going from bad to worse as children do not have an easy time during puberty and, if on top of that you hear voices, it will be twice as difficult. All things considered, it was time for some help, but that was not easy at this point either. We were referred to youth care, the waiting time was roughly ten months! How on earth can they help anybody (who is stuck) if you first have to wait for months? After the intake interview the whole family was put into therapy. That did not feel right. It made us feel very insecure and we got the feeling that we would not get much further with this. We gave up after a handful of sessions. All in all, a serious disappointment; you indicate that you need help (that is a pretty big step to take), then they let you wait ten months, only for you to discover that the care they are offering will only make things worse!

Around the age of 13, Tamsin went through a bad patch again and we found a therapist who worked according to the Prof Romme/Sandra Escher method. Tamsin started the treatment with a lot of confidence. We were wondering whether we would finally be successful in finding appropriate care. This was the first time that a therapist approached things from the right angle. However, her approach was too drastic after all. For Tamsin, it was very frightening. The therapist wanted to help her, but also to change her completely! Tamsin felt ill and scared when she had to go there (about two hours by car) and even more ill

on the way back – and that every Sunday!

The therapist taught her a great deal about herself, but she did not take Tamsin as a person sufficiently into account. I was not allowed to be present during the interviews and, within a short period, I would not recognise my own child anymore. She had to speak up for herself more and be more assertive. The approach was good, but Tamsin became increasingly scared, sad, quiet and did not want to change. She felt that, as a result, she would end up not being herself any more. I found it difficult to leave her there with the therapist. All along, I had made sure that Tamsin would be able to deal with her voices as well as possible and now there was someone who could possibly help, but she shut me out completely and scared Tamsin tremendously. I could only partly feel that letting go and trusting was supposed to be good for Tamsin. This time I did not take Tamsin by the hand to go home again, but the initiative came from her. She wrote a letter to the therapist saying that she would not be coming any more and why she would not come. She had made this decision on her own and she already had the letter ready when she told me that she wanted to quit. I was so proud of her; if that was not assertiveness then I do not know what is. I supported her decision and had the confidence that this girl would get there in the end. The letter was clear, honest and written with friendly words – assertive, but not attacking and that is how Tamsin wanted to be!

In hindsight I think that the therapist was generally right. However, the way in which she wanted to achieve it was not the right way for Tamsin at that moment. She has a strong character and, despite the voices, she remains true to herself. She does not want to change but do things her way and learn to deal with it. Tamsin is still a child that always adapts and I have never seen her get angry. However, we do see her change gradually, she has her own opinion and voices it more and more often. She gives you her well-thought-out opinion and is sweet and social, but also very clear. All in all someone you take into consideration, respect and, therefore, not always invisible any more.

At secondary school there were ups and downs for Tamsin. She started a 'bridging period' for the medium/higher level school and, the first two years, things went reasonably well. The third year was more difficult; the voices bothered her more at that point and she

became very insecure as a result. Going up from the third to the fourth grade was not possible, but she was able to switch from the third grade at the medium level school to the fourth grade of the lower level school. I had many reservations about that. Tamsin is clever enough to achieve the medium or higher level school and I feel that the lower level school is well below her abilities. I was afraid that she would sink even lower if there were no challenges at school any more as she needed these to get things done. However, Tamsin no longer wanted to. She was tired and insecure. In hindsight, the switch to the lower level school was not such a bad one after all. She was facing a couple of relaxing years ahead. She hardly had to make any effort at this school and still scored good grades. Moreover, she met her current boyfriend, Simon, and she fell in love.

In these years things were going well for Tamsin. She was not bothered by the voices that much and she enjoyed all the things around her. In those days, it became clear to Tamsin that she wanted to become a therapist helping children hearing voices. From our own experience we already knew that the current care system has very little to offer here. In order to achieve her objective, she had to go to medium level vocational college, since she did not attend the medium level (academic) school, in order to enrol for a polytechnic degree course. Tamsin started the SPW (social-pedagogic) course for an activities coach/trainer in Helmond, in the Netherlands. This is one of the first demand-led courses. It is a course that normally lasts four years, but because it is demand-led, it can be done in a shorter time too. You work at your own speed and the school supports students in this. So you are studying independently and the school helps and provides structure so that, at the end of the day, the students know what they are supposed to study and produce. Unfortunately things did not go as well as we had hoped. Since this teaching method was new to both the school and the teacher, there was a lack of any form of clarity and structure. The students did not have a clue at all about what was expected of them. Tamsin suffered a great deal from the voices, but also other physical problems. She felt insecure and sad. The voices were giving her a pretty rough time. She got eczema, bowel problems and, every now and then, she fainted, but she kept on going and fighting. At school, they saw a totally different Tamsin to the one we were used to

at home. In order to survive she regularly had to speak up for herself, this cost her a great deal of energy. Furthermore, she saw herself change and she was not happy with that. Her classmates saw a girl who could stand up for herself and respected and admired her for that, but Tamsin did not recognise herself any more and that made her insecure too and her physical symptoms were getting worse and worse.

At that time I also tried to support her as well as I could, so I started looking for help again. Via the website of the Resonance Association I found the email address of Sandra Esher. I passed it on to Tamsin and encouraged her to email Sandra. After several weeks of plucking up the courage, she emailed Mrs Esher. That is when the waiting started, would she email back? Every day emails were checked nervously. Sandra sent back a sweet and supportive email. Tamsin was happy and scared at the same time!

Through her email Sandra Esher gave Tamsin courage and she encouraged her to fill in the interview questionnaire and, in this way, work on her emotional recovery. This took up a lot of her energy, but she ploughed through it and spent many a difficult hour in front of the computer. When an email from Sandra arrived, it sometimes took a whole day before she could control her emotions and dared to open it. Responding to the emails and filling in the interview questionnaire was very difficult. Yet again I was very proud of Tamsin. On all fronts she was working on her recovery. Perhaps even more important was the fact that she did it in her own way. She was in a lot of pain, was constantly tired and insecure, but she was not going to give up. I witnessed it all and fought with her!

At school she stood up for herself; assertive, clear and also as non-confrontational as possible; she kept on asking for good support so that she could get her degree. Her eczema got worse and worse and inhibited her normal functioning and the voices kept on visiting her too. When she heard about the course 'Train the trainers for experience experts', led by Sandra Esher, she was 'umming and aahing' for a long time, but finally she requested information and enrolled for the course. Tamsin really wanted to do this course, since in the future she wanted to work with children hearing voices, so this was in preparation for her future job. Moreover, she thought it would be wonderful meeting Sandra Esher and to finally meet other voice hearers. She arranged

everything at school, so that she could do the course in school hours and had saved up for the course fee. I was happy that she started this course, but for totally different reasons than Tamsin's. Since things were not going well with her, I was very concerned. I saw the personal development of Tamsin and that made me really happy. However, Tamsin was still down. My expectations of the course were different to those of Tamsin. I had hoped that she would get to know people with whom she could identify and, in this way, get more insight into her own life too. So far we did not know any voice hearers and contact with fellow sufferers can be very positive. Moreover, I liked the fact that she would get to know Sandra Esher personally. Because of her article, I felt she would be helpful and I trusted my intuition. However, it was definitely the email contact between Sandra Esher and Tamsin which has been more helpful to us than all other therapists together. If Tamsin were to get more self-knowledge as a result of this course, it would be more than a success to me and worth its money.

Although we had both expected the course to be emotionally very difficult, unfortunately, participation in the course took up more energy than we had estimated, However, we had not expected that it would take up more energy than Tamsin had. She became sadder, quieter, had less and less energy (every night in bed by 8pm), could only go to school 20 per cent of the time and the eczema on her skin was so bad that, every now and then, she would faint because of the pain. Emotionally she was spent and there were days that she did not want to get out of bed any more and she definitely did not want to continue with the course. It hurts a lot to see your child like that and you cannot really help. I was sad too and emotionally not that stable any more. However, I was totally convinced that Tamsin had to continue this tough journey in order to get better at the end of it. I trusted my instincts again and forced Tamsin to continue with this course. For me, this was one of the most difficult things I ever had to do during the upbringing of my children. I would have loved to have taken my little girl into my arms to comfort her, but I had to put her on a train to the course and hope that she would be able to pull through.

On reflection this was a good decision. Tamsin showed her strength and perseverance and she finished the course. She sat in front of the computer for hours and hours to write her experience story, which

was so difficult. However, she managed and she wrote it and, as a result, she came to terms with many emotions and she has now dealt with them. She had already gained experience with filling in the interview questionnaire, but even that took up a lot of her perseverance. She learned a lot from the course!

She went through a phase of enormous personal development and I am now looking at a young adult with a great deal of self-knowledge, who is assertive in a clear, sweet way, who is social and who has faith in her future. No doubt there will be difficult times ahead in her life, but for the first time I have the feeling that I can let go of my girl and that she has the strength to enter adulthood by herself. I am so proud of Tamsin and have great respect for her as a person.

KARIN'S STORY

Anne is our only child. She is 13 years old now and, three years ago, she was plagued by two voices. As far as she can remember, Anne has been hearing voices from the age of six. In that year we moved to a different neighbourhood, but Anne remained at the same school, since it was a good school and she liked going there. She thought that the voices were friends who were all part of it. She was not bothered by them until the age of nine.

Anne was a sweet, happy baby. She did not cry a lot and was very easy. She is a very sensitive girl who had a paranormal gift. She picks up things that she simply cannot know. When she was small I did not really notice that very much. However, occasionally she said things that did not quite fit with her age. When the voices started to play up, the experiences happened more often and were more intense.

Personally, I sometimes had paranormal experiences too, particularly when I was younger, but they were different and not as frequent. I did not really think much about them either.

When Anne was three years old, I drove to the crèche at work with her and then suddenly from her child seat she said to me: 'I chose you as mummy and daddy'. Strange, just like that in front of the traffic light. I asked: 'What do you mean?' She said: 'It's simple, I just came up to you.'

Threat

When she was almost ten, she raised the alarm. One voice had become very malignant. The other voice would then take Anne's side. The voices scared and confused her. She was told to do or not to do certain things and she was threatened.

On the Internet I had been searching for more information about voice hearing, but you have to work through a load of rubbish before you find some serious information! I went to see our GP and he referred me to a child psychologist. We visited the RIAGG (Regional Institute for Mental Welfare) and were called up pretty quickly. An extensive intake procedure followed, during which everything was turned inside out, even us, the parents. I do not have pleasant memories about this. Anne was seen by a children's therapist who started to work on her self-confidence and resilience to make her stronger. They did games therapy. Anne liked going to the therapist who was very happy and extrovert. Anne bonded with her.

The voices threatened that they would hurt me, daddy or granny. They made her feel so scared that, even in the finest weather, she did not dare to go out. She was scared of everything. At the time she was suffering from many fits of anger. She would then break things in her room. She would do that when she was alone.

At school

Anne has always had a problem with maths. She is bad at it and she finds it very difficult to remember multiplication tables. Doing sums requires a lot of concentration that she cannot really manage for long. So when she really has to finish something, things don't go well.

At primary school, she was put in a special maths group and she did not like that. She did not like getting something wrong. I have tried to teach her that doing your best is good enough and that you cannot learn anything without making mistakes. She is good at languages and expressing herself. She reads a lot, at the moment she is devouring (girls') books so fast that I cannot imagine that she has really read everything. Her grade five teacher made a fool of her with maths and her classmates teased her about that. Anne only told me this during the summer holidays. The voices had become negative earlier, but not as bad as after the time the teacher had made a fool of her.

When Anne went up to grade six (she was ten at the time), she got a really nice, male teacher. I told him immediately about the voices and asked him to take that into consideration. He asked: 'Has she got a paranormal gift by any chance?' That response was a relief. He also mentioned that something like a complaints committee exists. We did not do anything with that information, however, we did talk to the headmaster at a later stage. During that first conversation, the teacher also said that he knew a woman who could help children with this type of problem, she had a gift. A while later he told me that he showed this woman a school photo of the entire class, without adding any comment. She immediately pointed at Anne and said: 'That child is going through a very tough time'.

Following that, developments happened in quick succession. Some events happened at the same time others crossed each other. The child psychologist wanted to do some tests regarding Anne's maths problem. I did not want that at the time, since Anne was having a hard enough time with the voices. However, the therapist insisted and she certainly had very good arguments in favour of tests, like: 'If you know what is wrong, there are appropriate solutions.' At school we discussed it with the team and the child therapist. The headmaster suggested that Anne could also follow maths one grade lower. I found that a good idea, in order to take off the pressure of maths. This worked, but in the end Anne was behind in maths and, at this point in time, we are still not quite sure how this is going to work out in her secondary school. It has probably influenced the advice she was given about which level of secondary school to go to next, but so be it. The fact that she is freed of the voices is far more important!

Confused

Anne indicated that, during that period, there were several moments that she did not want to live anymore. The voices made her life a living hell. 'Boze Moos' (angry Moos) was the worst. 'Boze Loos' (angry Loos) was in fact a positive voice which had always helped Anne, but recently it had 'defected' to the angry side, hence the name 'Boze Loos' (angry Loos). Often the voices would start a discussion amongst themselves. At these moments, it was very busy in Anne's head. She was never asleep before 11 o'clock at night. The voices would not let her sleep,

woke her up early and distracted her at school. Anne got confused and it was so bad that, at one point, she lost her grip on reality. She started getting delusions. She thought that I wanted to poison her. When I prepared food or drinks for her, I would take some of it myself in order to reassure her.

Then she believed that everybody was a robot apart from herself, even our little dog, since it had little green lights in its eyes. I was a robot too. You should have seen her. I was very shocked about this and I phoned the therapist. She explained that it was very comforting that within five minutes Anne had realised that she had been saying such strange things. I was to phone her if it happened again. She was talking about medication if things got worse.

Searching

The children's therapist was of the opinion that, if Anne became stronger and got more confidence, the role of the voices would diminish automatically. As a result of the work of the children's therapist, Anne indeed got a bit stronger, more positive, but the influence of the voices did not diminish. Anne never laughed.

Anne was really keen on telling her classmates what bothered her and she came up with the idea of holding a presentation for her class about it. I did not think it was such a good idea as not all of the children would understand it and she would then be teased about it. I did my utmost to talk her out of it and, if necessary, I would have forbidden her to do it. However, she told one or two children whom she was sure she could trust.

I made an appointment (without Anne) with the woman the teacher had mentioned to see who she was. She said she could help, but that, at the end of the day, Anne would still be left with a voice and that it would not be a supportive voice. I just did not want to accept that and started to search further.

More searching

Anne indicated that she really wanted to get in touch with a fellow sufferer. I thought of the studies of Marius Romme and Sandra Escher that I had read earlier. I thought: 'That woman simply has to know some children in our neighbourhood'. I was able to track down her email

address, mailed her and, to my surprise, she phoned me. I expressed my concern. We agreed that my husband, Anne and I would visit her at home, where she would conduct the interview for children hearing voices. The RIAGG had not done this. The result of the interview was that my husband acknowledged the extent of the problem, that he understood what it was like for Anne. Sandra wrote a short report about the interview which clearly mentioned Anne's experiences with the voices. I took this report to school as well as the RIAGG.

The visit to Sandra comforted me and helped me as a mother which was very important for me at the time. My husband found it difficult to cope with this issue. I found it hard to talk to him about it. Therefore, I had to go my own way here. In hindsight, his role in the whole story was very important. He stayed with both feet on the ground, remained positive and took care of many practical things that I found difficult. Furthermore, my sister and a very good friend provided me with both support and understanding.

Marius Romme had been present at the interview too and had said: 'The role of the voices cannot be reduced, as long as the voices control her life'. That had made me think. Something had to happen. I asked Sandra for telephone numbers of alternative counsellors who, she knew, had achieved good results. I phoned the one that was closest to me. Our first telephone contact did not feel that good and I could not face going there. Following that, I phoned Gieny van Landwijk in Nunhem. Gieny was very direct and promised that she could get rid of the voices. She told me that, although she did not really have time, she did not want a child to suffer that much. I was in the right place.

Gieny told Anne that the voices were not part of her, but she had quite a paranormal gift. She also said that Anne had not found her place on Earth, did not dare to do things, which had created an opening for the voices. During the first conversation, she and her partner Luigi (they worked together) showed what they were going to do. Some light classical music was played. Anne had to sit down with her eyes shut and with her little feet on the ground and Gieny said: 'A child that has not really found her place on Earth will get dizzy now'. Anne immediately got dizzy and felt like throwing up. Gieny is a 'no-nonsense' person. I liked her directness.

We visited once a week. A session did not take that long, but was very tiring. Anne had to close her eyes and be aware of herself. Anne could only describe this as: '… they would just come to me then, as I could see them'. Afterwards, we let her choose a lollipop as that helped with her energy levels. I was not allowed to be present at the sessions. Anne told me about them. She would tell me that Gieny and Luigi would hide behind a pillar (near Anne) to see what the voices would be doing. The voices got a real shock when they suddenly appeared. During our drive home from these sessions, Anne was in such good spirits.

Strange experiences

I found that Anne just had to continue with the children's therapist. Gieny said that that was OK, as long as she let go of the 'voices' subject whilst Gieny was working on that. I immediately talked to the therapist. She did not believe in my journey to spiritual healers (by the way, my husband did not either) but – thank goodness! – she would cooperate.

During that period, when I took Anne to bed once, she saw hands, coming from my back, holding her 'user manual'. She was scared that if people read that, she would be sent to prison. It was then that she also became scared of me. She was not able to explain the words 'user manual' in any more detail. Gieny probed further into this. Not long after, together with Anne, she put 'Boze Moos' in a very cramped prison so that he could not do any further damage. He had threatened to travel down to her heart and to make it stop beating. Together they had built a brick wall around the bars. The following week the wall fell down, but the bars survived.

There have been several of Anne's experiences where it seemed as if visionary things entered via the voice. However, the voice would distort it. The voice might shout that a murderer would appear, a world ruler who had helpers; Arsjraa or something like that. The voice was incredibly scared of this and would hide. This made Anne really scared too. It was at that point that she started getting confused. It was not until months later that, by coincidence, I stumbled upon the word 'Ashrayaa' on the Internet. I thought it sounded like it and I searched on. It turned out to be old Sanskrit and it meant 'protection'.

In that difficult period, I experienced the odd paranormal experience myself too. Once I heard footsteps late at night and I was

wondering what the neighbours were doing in the garage at this time. Then I realised that these were the footsteps of a child. I had a look upstairs, but Anne was asleep. I also heard footsteps upstairs at Gieny's while I was waiting in the corridor when she was busy upstairs with Anne. These were the footsteps of a man, so I assumed that these were Luigi (Gieny's partner), but it turned out that Luigi was not at home. Anne told me afterwards that, during the session whilst 'working', she had seen a dark figure on the landing. Anne would sometimes see images (silhouettes) at home too, sometimes dark ones, sometimes light.

The voices cannot do anything

Of course I knew the voices could not do anything to her. I would often tell her this, but for Anne it was totally different. The voices were (too) real.

After two months 'Boze Moos' was sent packing for good. We worked towards that moment. Just before, 'Boze Loos' had already left by himself. That voice listened to Anne again and at some point 'Boze Loos' asked: 'So what do you want me to do?' Anne answered: 'Well just pack your bags and never come back again.' The voice said: 'OK, I will leave now, ciao!' and that was the last thing she heard of that voice. Luigi did not react very enthusiastically. I understood, from him, that a voice like that should not start drifting. It should be discarded in the correct way.

The liberation

However, getting rid of 'Boze Moos' could only succeed if Anne really wanted it herself. Wanting it herself was very important. We had completely prepared for it and, at some point, Anne was ready. I was very tense at that most important moment. A new housekeeper who I did not know went upstairs with the telephone, right at the very moment that they were busy helping Anne. I wanted to grab her and pull her down the stairs. It was at that point that I thought: 'Karin, let go, this is not in your hands'.

The little cage of 'Boze Moos' was placed in a rocket and that rocket was sent to the moon. Anne saw the rocket getting smaller and smaller, until it became a little dot and disappeared out of sight. It had worked!

'Boze Moos' had left. This was an emotional moment and afterwards we were both very tired. Anne was allocated a little assistant on which she could fall back in the coming period. In her case, it was 'the blue moon'. She did indeed use her little assistant. Anne turned 11 the day after, but we did not celebrate. We just needed to recover from it all first. Anne did not dare to feel comfortable straightaway; for a while, she remained wary.

In the end Gieny and Luigi were able to help in nine sessions, whereas we had been going to the RIAGG for over a year by then. I let Anne continue with the children's therapist for a while, as it helped her at school.

Anne is more resilient now, not just mentally, but physically too. She took part in a resilience and self-defence course for girls between 12 and 15 years old. She had received a flyer at school. She was attracted by the words 'self-defence'. She did not like the first session as they had to hit things. However, once she finally managed to punch through her piece of wood, she was very proud and it gave her a real kick. She wanted nothing more than do the course again.

Anne was freed of the voices in the summer of 2007. By now, she had changed into a beautiful adolescent (she was 13) and was enjoying girly things. She is able to be herself again, she developed quite fast from that point onwards and when, after a long time, I heard a loud laugh for the first time again, I was so happy! Some friendly classmates found that Anne had changed a lot in a positive way; more open, positive and sweeter.

During her worst periods, Anne saw a lot of auras, in all kinds of colours and sizes. Later on, I never heard her mention these at all and I do not ask her about these either any more. It is only recently that it has started to happen again sporadically and, sometimes, Anne sees things about a person that she simply cannot know. I just leave it as it is, but she can always talk to me about this.

Setback

The things I personally found very difficult were the powerlessness, the despair, the invisibility of the enemy/imposter or whatever you call the thing which destroys your child. However, the support that I had wished for so desperately and even shouted for, came in the end

and I am very grateful for that! Accepting everything that happened will only be dealt with once you are allowed to look back.

When everything was over, I experienced quite a setback, in the second half of 2007. Earlier that year, I was overworked and that will have played a role too. Gieny could not help me at that time. I visited the RIAGG. After two months I had only had two conversations and I was still in the intake phase and had been crying there. I could not face continuing and I quit. They did not like that very much.

On the advice of a friend, I went to see a first-line psychologist (I did not know the difference at that time). He was available immediately and the only thing he asked was: 'What can I do for you?' I liked that and, as a result, a great deal came flowing out. He used beautiful metaphors in order to simplify things. I also wanted to know what a 'down-to-earth' psychologist thought about the voice-hearing phenomenon. His explanation, incidentally, did not help me any further. However, I was able to let things out and that was the purpose of it. I had to deal with it.

Occasionally I would also go and see a woman who had been mentioned by the teacher. This helped me a great deal as she was able to put her finger on the sore spot immediately. At the beginning of 2008, I suffered from a hernia. It was like my body was saying: 'So, now it is my turn again'. This lasted about seven months. What is truth? It is exactly what you perceive to be the truth.

Anne is looking forward to secondary school. She cannot remember everything about this awful period in her life.

References

Of course you can write a book full of advice, but people take advice more seriously if what you say has been published in books or peer-reviewed in academic journals. From the children's research the four articles below have been published in English and can be found on our website: www.hearing-voices.com.

Escher, A et al. (2002a) Independent course of childhood auditory hallucinations: A 3-year sequential follow-up study. *British Journal of Psychiatry, 181* (suppl. 43), s10–18.

Escher, A et al. (2002b) Formation of delusional ideation in adolescents hearing voices: A prospective study. *American Journal of Medical Genetics (Neuropsychiatric Genetics), 114*, 913–20.

Escher, A et al. (2003) Coping defence and depression in adolescents hearing voices. *Journal of Mental Health, 12* (1), 91–9.

Escher, A et al. (2004) Determinants of outcome in the pathways through care for children hearing voices. *International Journal of Social Welfare, 13*, 208–22.

Note from Sandra Escher: For my children's research I have been supported and advised by Prof. Marius Romme, Prof. Jim van Os, Prof. Phillip Delespaul, (Netherlands), Prof. Mervyn Morris, Prof. Richard Bentall and Prof. Phil Thomas (United Kingdom). I am very grateful for their help.

LITERATURE USED IN THE RESEARCH

Achenbach, TM (1991) Manual for the Child Behavior Checklist (CBCL)/4–18 and 1991 profiles. Burlington,VT: University of Vermont, Department of Psychiatry.

Agar, J, Argyle, N & Aderholds, V (2003) Sexual and physical abuse during childhood and adulthood as predictors of hallucinations, delusions and thought disorder. *Psychology and Psychotherapy: Theory, Research and Practice, 76*, 1–22.

Al-Issa, I (1977) Social and cultural aspects of hallucinations. *Psychological Bulletin, 84* (3), 570–87.

Al-Issa, I (1978) Sociocultural factors in hallucinations. *International Journal of Social Psychiatry, 24*, 167–76.

Allan, JG & Goyne, L (1995) Dissociation and vulnerability to psychotic experiences. The Dissociative Experience Scale and the MMP1-2. *Journal of Nervous and Mental Disease, 183*, 615–22.

Alschulzer, A (1997) The world of the inner voice. Unpublished data in Heery, MW (1993) Inner voice experiences. In: M Romme & A Escher (eds) *Accepting Voices*. London: Mind.

Altmann, H, Collins, M & Mundy, P (1997) Subclinical hallucinations and delusions in nonpsychotic adolescents. *Journal of Child Psychology and Psychiatry, 38* (4),413–20.

American Psychiatric Association (1980) *Diagnostic and Statistical Manual of Mental Disorders* (3rd edn). Washington DC: APA.

Andrade, C & Srinath, S (1986) The auditory hallucinations and smaller superior temporal gyral volume in schizophrenia. *American Journal of Psychiatry, 147*, 1457–62.

Andreasen, NC (1997) *Our Brave New World. Anatomische les.* Amsterdam: de Volkskrant.

Bak, M, Van der Spil, F, Gunther, N et al. (2001) Macs II. Does coping enhance subjective control over symptoms? *Acta Psychiatrica Scandinavia, 103*, 460–4.

Bak, M, Van der Spil, F, Gunter, N, Radstaske, S, Delespaul, P & van Os, J (2001) MACS-I. Maastricht Assessment of coping stategies: A brief instrument to assess coping with psychotic symptoms. *Acta Psychiatrica Scandinavia, 103*, 543–59.

Barnes, TR, Curson, DA, Liddle, PF & Patel, M (1989) The nature of the prevalence of depression in chronic schizophrenic in-patients. *British Journal of Psychiatry, 154*, 486–91.

Barrett, TR & Etheridge, JB (1992) Verbal hallucinations in normals 1: People who hear 'voices'. *Applied Cognitive Psychology, 6*, 379–87.

Barta, PE, Pearlson, GD & Powers, RE (1990) Auditory hallucinations and smaller superior temporal gyral volume in schizophrenia. *American Journal of Psychiatry, 147*, 1457–62.

Beck, AT (1952) Successful out-patient psychotherapy of a chronic schizophrenic with a delusion based on borrowed guilt. *Psychiatry, 15*, 305–12

Bender, L (1970) *The Maturation Process and Hallucinations in Children. Origin and mechanism of hallucinations.* W Kemp (ed). New York: Plenum.

Bender, L & Lipkowitz, HH (1940) Hallucinations in children. *American Journal of Orthopsychiatry.* New York: Plenum.

Bernstein, EM & Putman, FW (1986) Development, reliability and validity of a dissociation scale (DES). *Journal of Nervous and Mental Disease, 174*, 727–35.

Bentall, RP (ed) (1990) *Reconstructing Schizophrenia.* London/New York: Routledge.

Bentall, RP (2003) *Madness Explained: Psychosis and human nature.* London: Penguin.

Bentall, RP, Haddock, G & Slade, PD (1994) Cognitive behavioural therapy for persistent auditory hallucinations. *Behavioural Therapy, 25*, 51–66.

Bentall, RP, Jackson, HF & Pilgrim, D (1988) Abandoning the concept of 'Schizophrenia': Some implications of validity arguments for psychological research into psychotic phenomena. *British Journal of Clinical Psychology, 66*, 493–9.

Bentall, RP & Lowe, CF (1987) The role of verbal behaviour in human learning III: Instrumental effects in children. *Journal of the Experimental Analysis of Behaviour, 47*, 177–90.

Bentall, RP, Lowe, CF & Beasty, A (1985) The role of verbal behaviour in human learning

II: Developmental differences. *Journal of the Experimental Anaysis of Behaviour, 3*, 165–81.

Bentall, RP & Slade, PD (1985) Reality testing in auditory hallucinations: A signal detection analysis. *British Journal of Clinical Psychology, 24*, 159–69.

Bentall, RP & Slade, PD (1986) Verbal hallucinations, unintendedness and the validity of the schizophrenic diagnosis. *The Behavioral and Brain Science, 9*, 519–20.

Berrios, GE & Bulbena, A (1987) Post psychotic depression: The Fulbourn cohort. *Acta Psychiatrica Scandinavia, 76*, 89–93.

Bertalanffy, L von (1950) An outline of general system theory. *British Journal of Science, 1* (2), 134–65.

Berteaux, D (ed.) (1981) *Biography and Society: The life history approach in the social sciences.* Beverly Hills, CA: Sage Publications.

Bettes, BA & Walker, E (1987) Positive and negative symptoms in psychotic and other psychiatrically disturbed children. *Journal of Child Psychology and Psychiatry, 28* (4), 555–68.

Bijl, RV, Ravelli, A & van Zessen, G (1998) Prevalence of psychotic disorder in the general population: Results from The Netherlands mental health survey and incidence study. *Social Psychiatry Epidemology, 33*, 587–96.

Birchwood, M & Chadwick, P (1997) The omnipotence of voices: Testing the validity of a cognitive model. *Psychological Medicine, 27*, 1345–53.

Birchwood, M, Meaden, A, Tower, P et al. (2000) The power and omnipotence of voices: Subordination and entrapment by voices and significant others. *Psychological Medicine, 30*, 337–44.

Bleuler, E (1911) *Dementia Preacox or the Group of Schizophrenias.* (Trans J Zinkin. International University Press, New York, 1950.) Leipzig: Deuticke.

Bleuler, M (1978) *Die Schizophrenen geistestoringen im lichte langjahriger kranken und familen geschichten.* [Schizophrenic Disorders: Long-term patient and family studies.] (Trans SM Clemens. Stuttgart: Thieme, 1972.) New Haven and London: Yale University Press.

Blom, JD (2003) *Deconstructing Schizophrenia: An analysis of the epistemic and nonepistemic values that govern the biomedical schizophrenia concept.* Amsterdam: Boom.

Boevink, W & Escher, S (2001) *Zelfverwonding begrijpelijk maken.* Bemelen, The Netherlands: St. Positieve Gezondheidszorg.

Boker, W, Brenner, HD, Gestner, G, Keller, F, Muller, J & Spichtig, L (1984) Self-healing strategies amoung schizophrenics: Attemps at compensation for basic disorders. *Acta Psychiatrica Scandinavia, 69*, 373–8.

Boon, S & Draijer, N(1990) Dissociative disorders in the Netherlands: a clinical investigation of 65 patients. In: BG Braun & EB Carlson. *Dissociative Disorders: Proceedings of the 8th international conference on multiple personality/ dissociative states.* Chicago: Rush.

Bosga, D (1993) Parapsychology and hearing voices. In: M Romme & A Escher (eds), *Accepting Voices.* London: Mind, pp 106–12.

Bourguignon, E (1970) Hallucination and trance: An antropologist's perspective. In: W Kemp (ed), *Origin and Mechanism of Hallucinations.* New York: Plenum.

Boyle, M (1990) *Schizophrenia – A scientific delusion?* London/New York: Routledge.

Bracken, P & Thomas, P (2000) Cognitive therapy, Cartesianism and the moral order. *European Journal of Psychotherapy, Counselling and Health, 2,* 325–44.

Bracken, P & Thomas, P (2004) Postpsychiatry: A new direction for mental health. *British Medical Journal, 322,* 724–7.

Brand, M (1986) Intended versus intentional action. *Behavioral and Brain Science, 9,* 520–1.

Brebion, G, Amador, X, David, A, Malaspina, D & Sharif, Z (2000) Positive symptomatology and source monitoring failure in schizophrenia: An analysis of symtom-specific effects. *Psychiatry Research, 95,* 119–31.

Breier, A & Strauss, JS (1983) Self-control in psychotic disorders. *Archives of General Psychiatry, 40* (10), 1141–5.

Brenner, HD, Boker, W, Muller, J, Spichtig, L &Wurgler, S (1987) On autoprotective efforts of schizophrenics, neurotics and controls. *Acta Psychiatrica Scandinavia, 75,* 405–14.

Burritt, I (1991) Social relations, culture and the self. In: *Social Selves: Theories of the social formation of personality.* London: International Society for Environmental Ethics, pp 137–58.

Carter, DM, Mackinnon, A & Copolov, DL (1996) Patients' strategies for coping with auditory hallucinations. *The Journal of Nevous and Mental Disease, 184* (3), 159–64

Chadwick, P & Birchwood, M (1994) The omnipotence of voices: A cognitive approach to auditory hallucinations. *British Journal of Psychiatry, 164,* 190–201.

Chadwick, PDJ & Birchwood, MJ (1995) The omnipotence of voices II: The beliefs about voices questionnaire. *British Journal of Psychiatry, 165,* 773–6.

Chambers, WJ, Puig-Antich, J, Tabrizi, MA & Davies, M (1982) Psychotic symptoms in prepuberal depressive disorder. *Archives of General Psychiatry, 39* (8), 921–7.

Ciompi, L (1980) The natural history of schizophrenia in the long term. *British Journal of Psychiatry, 136,* 413–20.

Cohen, CI & Berk, LA (1985) Personal coping styles of schizophrenic outpatients. *Hospital and Community Psychiatry, 36* (4), 407–10.

Coleman, R (1999) *Recovery: An alien concept.* Gloucester: Handsell Publishing.

Clayton, D & Hills, M (1993) Cox's regression models. In: *Statistical Methods in Epidemiology.* Oxford: Oxford University Press, pp 298–306.

Cleghorn, JM, Franco, S & Szechtman, B (1992) Towards a brain map of auditory hallucinations. *American Journal of Psychiatry, 149,* 1062–9.

Cole, M & Cole, SR (1989) *The Development of Children.* New York: Scientific American.

Culberg, J & Nybäck, H (1992) Persistent auditory hallucinations correlate with the size of the third ventricle in schizophrenic patients. *Acta Psychioatrica Scandinavia, 86,* 469–72.

Del Beccaro, MA, Burke, P & McCauley, E (1988) Hallucinations in children: A follow-up study. *Journal of the American Academy of Child and Adolescent Psychiatry, 27,* 462–5.

Despert, JL (1948) Delusional and hallucinatory experiences in children. *The American Journal of Psychiatry, 104* (8), 528–37.

Eaton, WW, Romanonski, A, Anthony, JC et al. (1991) Screening for psychosis in the general population with a self-report interview. *Journal of Nervous and Mental Disease, 179,* 689–93.

Ensink, B (1992) *Confusing Realities: A study on childhood sexual abuse and psychiatric*

symptoms. Amsterdam: VU University Press.

Ensink, B (1993) Trauma: A study of child abuse and hallucinations. In: M Romme & S Escher (eds), *Accepting Voices*. London: Mind.

Escher, A, Romme, M (1998) Small talk: Voice-hearing in children. *Open Mind*, July/August.

Escher, A, Romme, M, Buiks, A, Delespaul, P & van Os, J (2002a) Independent course of childhood auditory hallucinations: A sequential 3-year follow-up study. *British Journal of Psychiatry, 181* (suppl. 43), s10–18

Escher, A, Romme, M, Buiks, A, Delespaul, P & van Os, J (2002b) Formation of delusional ideation in adolescents hearing voices: A prospective study. *American Journal of Medical Genetics, 114*, 913–20.

Escher, A, Delespaul, P, Romme, M, Buiks, A & van Os, J (2003) Coping defence and depression in adolescents hearing voices. *Journal of Mental Health, 12* (1), 91–9.

Escher, A, Morris, M, Buiks, A, Delespaul, P, van Os, J & Romme, M (2004) Determinants of outcome in the pathways through care for children hearing voices. *International Journal of Social Welfare, 13*, 208–22.

Esquirol, JED (1832) Sur les illusions des sens chez les aliénes. *Archives Général de Médicine, 2*, 5–23.

Famularo, R, Kinscherff, R & Fenton, T (1992) Psychiatric diagnoses of maltreated children: Preliminary findings. *Journal of American Academic Child Adolescents Psychiatry, 31*, 863–7.

Falloon, IR & Talbot, RE (1981) Persistent auditory hallucinations: Coping mechanisms and implications for management. *Psychological Medicine, 11*, 329–39.

Feinberg, I (1970) Hallucinations, dreaming and rem sleep. In: W Kemp (ed), *Origins and Mechanisms of Hallucinations*. New York/London: Plenum Press, pp 125–32.

Fennig, S, Susser, ES, Pilowsky, DJ et al. (1997) Childhood hallucinations preceding the first psychotic episode. *Journal of Nervous and Mental Disease, 185*, 115–17.

Flavell, JH, Miller, PH & Scott, M (1993) *Cognitive Development* (third edition). New Jersey: Prentice Hall.

Foley, MA, Johnson, MK, & Ray, CL (1983) Age-related changes in confusion between memories for thoughts and memories for speech. *Child Development, 54*, 51–60.

Foster, DA & Caplan, RD (1994) Cognitive influences on perceived change in social support, motivation, and symptoms of depression. *Applied Cognitive Psychology, 8*, 123–39.

Frith, CD (1979) Conscious information processing and schizophrenia. *British Journal of Psychiatry, 134*, 225–35.

Frith, C (1992) *The Cognitive Neuropsychology of Schizophrenia*. Hove, UK, and Hillsdale, NJ: Lawrence Erlbaum Associates.

Freud, S (1917/1957) *Metapsychological Supplement to the Theory of Dreams* (Standard Edition). London: Hogarth Press, 217–35.

Freud, S (1923/1927) *The Ego and Id*. London: Hogarth Press.

Galdos, PM, van Os, JJ & Murray, RM (1993) Puberty and the onset of psychosis. *Schizophrenia Research, 10* (1), 7–14.

Galdos, PM & van Os, JJ (1995). Gender, psychopathology and development from puberty to early childhood. *Schizophrenia Research, 14* (2), 105–12.

Garralda, ME (1984a) Psychotic children with hallucinations. *British Journal of Psychiatry, 145*, 74–7.

Garralda, ME (1984b) Hallucinations in children with conduct and emotional disorder: 1. The clinical phenomena. *Psychological Medicine*, *14*, 589–96.

Glaser, B & Strauss, A (1967) *The Discovery of Grounded Theory: Strategies for qualitative research*. New York: Aldine de Gruyter, p 45.

Goff, DC, Brotman, AW, Kindlon, D et al. (1991) Self-reports of childhood abuse in chronically psychotic patients. *Psychiatry Research, 37*, 73–80.

Golomb, C & Galasso, L (1995) Make belief and reality: Explorations of imaginary realm. *Developmental Psychology, 31* (5), 800–10.

Green, EL et al. (1973) Some methods of evaluating behavioral variations in children 6 to 18. *Journal of the American Academy of Child Psychiatry, 12* (3), 531–53.

Green, P & Preston, M (1981) Reinforcement of vocal correlates of auditory hallucinations by auditory feedback: A case study. *British Journal of Psychiatry, 139*, 204–8.

Green, WH, Padron-Gayol, M, Hardesty, AS & Bassiri, M (1992) Schizophrenia with childhood onset: A phenomenological study of 38 cases. *Journal of American Academic Child and Adolescent Psychiatry, 31* (5), 968–76.

Greenbaum, PE & Dedrick, RF (1998) Hierarchical conformation factor analysis of the child behaviour checklist 4–18. *Psychological Assessment, 10*, 149–55.

Haddock, G & Slade, PD (1996) *Cognitive Behavioral Interventions with Psychotic Disorders*. London: Routledge.

Hammersley, P, Dias, A, Todd, G, Bowen-Jones, K, Reilly, B & Bentall, RP (2003) Childhood trauma and hallucinations in bipolar affective disorder: A preliminary investigation. *British Journal of Psychiatry, 182*, 543–7.

Harris, PL, Brown, E, Marriott, C et al. (1991) Monsters, ghosts and witches: Testing limits of fantasy-reality distinction in young children. *British Journal of Developmental Psychology, 9*, 105–23.

Hart de Ruyter, T & Kamp, LNJ (1973) *Hoofdlijnen van de kinderpsychiatrie*. Deventer: Van Lochem Slaterus.

Hartman, CA, Hox, J, Auerbach, J et al. (1999) Syndrome dimensions of the child behaviour checklist and the teacher report form: A critical empirical evaluation. *Journal of Child Psychology and Psychiatry and Allied Disciplines, 40*, 1095–116.

Heilbrun, AB, Blum, N & Haas, M (1983) Cognitive vulnerability to auditory hallucinations. *British Journal of Psychiatry, 143*, 294–9.

Herman, J (1997) *Trauma and Recovery: The aftermath of violence – from domestic abuse to political terror*. New York: Basic Books.

Hoffman, RE (1986) Verbal hallucinations and language production processes in schizophrenia. *Behavioural and Brian Science, 9*, 503–48.

Honig, A, Romme, MAJ, Ensink, B, Escher, S, Pennings, M & de Vries, M (1998) Auditory hallucinations: A comparison between patients and nonpatients. *Journal of Nervous and Mental Disease, 186*, 646–51.

Hoofdakker, RH van den (1995) *De mens als speelgoed*. Houten: Bohn Stafleu van Loghum.

Inouye, T & Shimizu, A (1970) The electromyografic study of verbal hallucination. *Journal of Nervous and Mental Disease, 151*, 415–22.

Jenner, A, Monteiro, ACD, Zargo-Cardoso, JA & Cunha-Oliveira, JA (1993) *Schizophrenia: A disease or some ways of being human*. Sheffield: Sheffield Academic Press.

Jong, M de (1997) *60 Ways to Drop your Client*. [Het anti-participatie boekje.] Utrecht: Netwerk clientdeskundigen NP/CG.

Kemph, JP (1987) Hallucinations in psychotic children. *Journal of American Academic Child and Adolescence Psychiatry*, *26* (4), 556–9.

Kendler, KS, McGuire, M, Gruenberg, AM et al. (1994) Clinical heterogeneity in schizophrenia and the pattern of psychopathology in relatives: Results from a epidemiologically based family study. *Acta Psychiatrica Scandinavia*, *89*, 294–300.

Kingdon, D & Turkington, D (1991) A role for cognitive-behavioral strategies in schizophrenia. *Social Psychiatry and Psychiatric Epidemiology*, *26*, 101–3.

Kingdon, DG and Turkington, D (1994) *Cognitive-behavioural Therapy of Schizophrenia*. Hove: Laurence Erlbaum Associates.

Kingdon, D & Turkington, D (eds) (2003) *The Case Study Guide to Cognitive Behavioural Therapy of Psychosis*. Hoboken, NJ: John Wiley & Sons.

Kleinman, A (1988) *Rethinking Psychiatry from Cultural Category to Personal Experience*. New York: The Free Press.

Kospodoulus, S, Kaninsberg, J, Côté, A & Fiedorowicz, C (1987) Hallucinatory experiences in nonpsychotic children. *Journal of American Academic Child and Adolescent Psychiatry*, *26* (3), 373–80.

Kreapelin, E (1883) *Compendium der Psychiatrie. Zum Gebrauche fur Studirende and Arzte*. Leipzig: Verlag von Johann Ambrosius Abel.

Kreapelin, E (1913) *Psychiatrie, ein Lehrbuch fur Studerende und Artzt*. [Psychiatry, a textbook for students and practitioners] (8th edn, vol 3.) Leipzig: Barth.

Lazarus, RS & Folkman, S (1984) *Stress, Apprisal and Coping*. New York: Springer Verlag.

Leff, J (1988) *Psychiatry Around the Globe: A transcultural view*. New York: Dekker.

Leudar, I, Thomas, P, McNally, D & Glinski, A (1977) What voices can do with words: Pragmatics of verbal hallucinations. *Psychological Medicine*, *27*, 885–97.

Leudar, I & Thomas, P (2000) *Voices of Reason, Voices of Insanity. Studies of verbal hallucinations*. London and Philadephia: Routledge.

Linville, PW (1987) Self-complexity as a cognitive buffer against stress-related illness and depression. *Journal of Personality and Social Psychology*, *52* (4), 663–76.

Lukoff, D, Neuchterlein, KH & Ventura, J (1986) Manual for expanded Brief Psychiatric Rating Scale. *Schizophrenia Bulletin*, *12*, 594–602.

McGee, R, Williams, S & Poulton, R (2000) Hallucinations in non-psychotic children (letter). *Journal of American Academic Child and Adolescent Psychiatry*, *39* (1), 12–13.

McGuigan, FJ (1996) Covert oral behaviour and auditory hallucinations. *Psychophysiology*, *3*, 73–80.

McGuire, PK, Shah, GMS & Murray, RM (1993) Increased blood flow in Broca's area during auditory hallucinations. *Lancet*, *342*, 703–6.

Miller, JG (1967) General system theory, In: A Freedman (ed), *Comprehensive Textbook of Psychiatry*. Baltimore: Williams & Wilkins Co.

Mintz, A & Alpert,M (1972) Imaginary vividness, reality testing and schizophrenic hallucinations. *Journal of Abnormal Psychology*, *79* (3), 310–16.

Mueser, KT, Valentiner, DP & Agresta, J (1997) Coping with negative symptoms of schizophrenia: Patient and family perspectives. *Schizophrenia Bulletin*, *23*, 329–39.

Musalek, M, Podreka, L, Walter, H et al. (1989) Auditory hallucinations, tactile hallucinations and normal controls. *Comprehensive Psychiatry*, *30* (1), 99–108

O'Hagan, M (1993) *Stopovers on My Way Home from Mars*. London: Survivors Speak Out.

Overall, JE & Gorham, D (1962) The Brief Psychiatric Rating Scale. *Psychological Reports*, *10*, 799–812.

Pennings, M & Romme, M (1996) Stemmen horen bij schizofrene patienten, patienten met een dissociatieve stoornis en niet-patienten. In: M de Hert et al. (eds), *Zin in Waanzin*. Amsterdam: Babylon-de Geus, pp 127–40.

Piaget, J (1974) *The Child and Reality*. London: Muller.

Polanyi, L (1985) *Telling the American Story: A structural and cultural analysis of conversational storytelling*. Norwood, NJ: Ablex.

Pope, CA & Kwapil, TR (2000) Dissociative experiences in hypothetically psychosis-prone college students. *Journal of Nervous and Mental Disease*, *188*, 530–6.

Posey, TB & Losch, ME (1983) Auditory hallucinations of hearing voices in 375 normal subjects. *Imagination, Cognition and Personality*, *3* (2), 99–113.

Posey, TB (1986) Verbal hallucinations also occur in normals. *Behavioural and Brain Sciences*, *9*, 530.

Poulton, R, Caspi, A, Moffit, TE, Cannon, M, Murray, R & Harrington, H (2000) Children's self-reported psychotic symptoms and adult schizophreniform disorder: A 15-year longitudinal study. *Archives of General Psychiatry*, *17* (11), 1053–8.

Praag, HM van (1993) *Make-believes in Psychiatry or The Perils of Progress*. New York: Brunner/Mazel.

Pruett, KD (1984) A chronology of defensive adaptations to severe psychological trauma. *Psychoanalytic Study of the Child*, *39*, 591–612.

Putman, FW & Peterson, G (1994) Further validation of the child dissociative checklist. *Dissociation*, *7*, 204–20.

Rabkin, R (1970) Do you see things that aren't there? Construct validity of the concept of 'hallucinations'. In: W Kemp (ed), *Origins and Mechanisms of Hallucinations*. New York, London: Plenum Press, pp 112–24.

Rankin, P & O'Carrol, P (1995) Reality monitoring and signal detection in individuals prone to hallucinations. *British Journal of Clinical Psychology*, *34*, 517–28.

Read, J & Reynolds, J (1996) *Speaking our Minds: An anthology of personal experiences and its consequences*. London: The Open University/Macmillan.

Robins, LN, Wing. J, Wittchen, HU et al. (1988) The Composite International Diagnostic Interview: An epidemiologic instrument suitable for use in cogjunction with different diagnostic systems and in different cultures. *Arch Gen Psychiatry*, *45*, 1069–77.

Romme, MAJ (1996) *Understanding Voices*. Gloucester: Handsell Publications.

Romme, MAJ & Escher, ADMAC (1989) Hearing voices. *Schizophrenia Bulletin*, *15* (2), 209–16.

Romme, MAJ & Escher, ADMAC (1993) *Accepting voices*. London: Mind.

Romme, MAJ & Escher, ADMAC (1996) Empowering people who hear voices. In: *Cognitive Behavioural Interventions with Psychotic Disorders*. London: Routledge, pp 137–50.

Romme, MAJ & Escher, ADMAC (2000) *Making Sense of Voices*. London: Mind.

Romme, MAJ, Honig, A, Noorthoorn, O & Escher, ADMAC (1992) Coping with voices: An emancipatory approach. *British Journal of Psychiatry*, *161*, 99–103.

Romme, MAJ, Kraan, H & Rotteveel, R (1981) *Wat is sociale Psychiatrie?* [What is social psychiatry?] Alphen aan den Rijn/Brussels: Samson Uitgeverij.

Ross, CA, Anderson, G & Clark, P (1994) Childhood abuse and the positive symptoms of schizophrenia. *Hospital and Community Psychiatry*, *42*, 489–91.

Ross, CA & Pam, A (1995) *Pseudo Science in Biological Psychiatry: Blaming the body.* London: Wiley.

Rothstein, A (1981) Hallucinatory phenomena in childhood. *Journal of the American Academy of Child Psychiatry*, *20*, 623–5.

Routledge (2000) *Routledge Encyclopedia of Philosophy.* London: Routledge.

Rund, BR (1986) Verbal hallucinations and information processing. *Behavioral and Brain Science*, *9*, 531–2.

Ryan, ND, Puig-Antich, J, Ambrosini, H, Robbinson, D, Nelson, B, Lyengar, S & Twomey, J (1987) The clinical picture of major depression in children and adolescents. *Archives of General Psychiatry*, *44* (10), 854–61.

Schneider, K (1949/1974) The concept of delusion. (Trans H.Marchall) In: SR Hirch & M Shepherd (eds), *Themes and Variations in European Psychiatry.* Bristol: John Wright & Sons, pp 33–9.

Schneider, K (1959) *Clinical Psychopathology* (5th edn). New York: Grune & Stratton.

Schreier, HA, (1998) Auditory hallucinations in nonpsychotic children with affective syndroms and migraines: Report of 13 cases (see comments). *Journal of Child Neurology*, *13* (8), 377–82.

Shaffer, D, Gould, MS, Brasic, J, Ambrosini, P, Fisher, P, Bird, H & Aluwahlie, S (1983) A children's global assessment scale (CGAS). *Archives of General Psychiatry*, *40* (11), 1228–31.

Sidgewick, HA et al. (1894) Report of the census of hallucinations. *Proceedings of the Society of Psychiatric Research*, *26*, 259–394.

Simonds, JF (1975) Hallucinations in nonpsychotic children and adolescents. *Journal of Youth and Adolescence*, *4* (20), 171–82.

Singer, J (1973) *The Child's World of Make Believe: Experimental studies of imaginative play.* New York: Academic Press.

Slade, PD (1976) An investigation of psychological factors involved in predisposition to auditory hallucinations. *Psychological Medicine, 6,* 123–32.

Slade, PD & Bentall, RP (1988) *Sensory Deception: A scientific analysis of hallucinations.* London: Croom Helm Ltd.

Spitzer, C, Haug, HJ & Freyberger, HJ (1977) Dissociative symptoms in schizophrenic patients with positive and negative symptoms. *Psychopathology*, *30*, 67–75.

STATA Corporation (1999) *STATA Statistical Software Release 6.0.* College Station, TX: STATA Corporation.

Tarrier, N (1987) An investigation of residual psychotic symptoms in discharged schizophrenic patients. *British Journal of Clinical Psychology*, *26*, 141–3.

Tarrier, N, Beckett, R, Harwood, S, Baker, A, Yusupoff, L & Ugarteburu, I (1993) A trial of two cognitive-behavioural methods of treating drug-resistant residual psychotic symptoms in schizophrenic patients: I. Outcome. *British Journal of Psychiatry*, *162*, 524–32.

Taylor, M, Carthwright, BS & Carslon, SM (1993) A developmental investigation of children's imaginary companions. *Developmental Psychology*, *29* (2), 276–85.

Thomas, P (1997) *The Dialectics of Schizophrenia.* London/New York: Free Association.

Thomas, P, Bracken, P & Leudar, I (2004) Hearing voices: A phenomenological-hermeneutic approach. *Cognitive Neuropsychiatry*, *9*, 13–23.

Thomas, P & Bracken, P (2004) Critical psychiatry in practice. *Advances in Psychiatric Treatment*, *10*, 361–70.

Tien, AY (1991) Distributions of hallucination in the population. *Social Psychiatry and Psychiatric Epidemiology*, *26*, 287–92.

Timimi, S (2002) *Pathological Child Psychiatry and Medicalisation of Childhood*. London: Brunner-Routledge.

Topor, A (2001) *Managing Contradictions: Recovery from severe mental disorders*. Edsbruk, Sweden: Akademitryck AB.

van Os, J, Hanssen, M, Bijl, R-V & Ravelli, A (2000) Straus (1969) revisited: A psychosis continuum in the general population? *Schizophrenia Research*, *45*, 11–20.

van Os, J & McKenna, P (2003) *Does Schizophrenia Exist?* (Maudsley Discussion Paper no. 12). London: Institute of Psychiatry Media Support Unit.

van Os, J, Verdoux, H, Maurice-Tison, S, Gay, B, Liraud, F, Salamon, R & Bourgeois, M (1999) Self-reported psychosis-like symptoms and the continuun of psychosis. *Social Psychiatry Psychiatric Epidemiology*, *34*, 459–63.

Ventura, J, Green, MF, Shaner, A et al. (1993) Training and quality assurance with the Brief Psychiatric Rating Scale (BPRS): The drift busters. *International Journal of Methods in Psychiatric Research*, *3*, 221–4.

Ventura, J, Ludoff, D, Neuchterlein, PR, Green, MF & Shaner, A (1993) Brief Psychiatric Rating Scale (BPRS) expanded version: Scales, anchor points and administration manual. *International Journal of Methods in Psychiatric Research*, *3*, 227–44.

Verdoux, H, van Os, J, Maurice-Tison, S, Gay, B, Salamon, R & Bourgeois, ML (1999) Increased accurence of depression in psychosis-prone subjects: A follow-up study in primary care setting. *Comprehensive Psychiatry*, *40*, 462–8.

Verhulst, FC (1992) *Kinder en jeugdpsychiatrie*. Assen/Maastricht: Van Gorcum.

Verhulst, FC, Van der Ende, J & Koot, HMH et al. (1996) Handleiding voor de CBCL 4–18: Sopia Kinderziekenhuis/Academisch Ziekenhuis, Erasmus Universiteit.

Vygotsky, LSV (1962) *Thought and Language*. Cambridge, MA: MIT Press.

Warner, R. (1994) *Recovery from Schizophrenia: Psychiatry and political economy*. London: Routledge.

Watson, J (1998) *Hearing Voices: A common human experience*. Melbourne: Hill of Content.

Wenar, C (1994) *Developmental Psychopathology: From infancy through adolescence* (third edition). New York: McGraw-Hill.

West, DE (1948) A mass observation questionnaire on hallucinations. *Journal of the Society for Psychical Research*, *34,* 187–96.

Winkler Prins (2002) *Encyclopedia*. Winkler Prins, Netherlands.

Yeates, TT & Bernnard, JR (1988) The 'haunted' child: Grief, hallucinations and family dynamics. *Journal of the American Academy of Child and Adolescent Psychiatry*, *27* (5), 573–81.

Young, HF, Bentall, RP, Slade, PD & Dewey, ME (1986) Disposition towards hallucination, gender and EPQ score: A brief report. *Personality and Individual Differences*, *7* (2), 247–9.

Zilboorg, G & Henry, GW (1941) *A History of Medical Psychology*. New York: Norton.